THE WELLSPRING

THE WELLSPRING

A GUIDE TO DELIVERING HEALING SPACES IN CALIFORNIA

BRIAN B. JONES

Brian B. Jones
The Wellspring
A Guide to Delivering Healing Spaces in California

Published by Spines Publishing Platform
ISBN: 979-8-90002-236-9

Spines

CONTENTS

Welcome to "The Wellspring" vii
Introduction ix
A Note from the Author xi

PART ONE
SETTING THE VISION

1. Foundations of Behavioral Health Real Estate Development 3
2. Strategic Planning and Feasibility Analysis 25
3. Team Assembly and Leadership Structure 53
4. The Owner's Advisor, Strategic Leadership 69
5. Financing Behavioral Health Infrastructure 81

PART TWO
FROM CONCEPT THRU PERMITTING

6. Site Selection: Laying the Groundwork for Success 91
7. Stakeholder Support 105
8. Facility Programming and Conceptual Design 119
9. Best Practices for Behavioral Health Care Design 133
10. Entitlements, Permitting, and Approvals 157

PART THREE
ACCELERATION, TALENT, EXCELLENCE

11. Best Practices of Successful Behavioral Health Real Estate Development 167
12. Advanced strategies for accelerating behavioral health facility delivery while maintaining quality and compliance standards 189
13. "25 Experts on the Development Team: The Power of Expertise" 207
14. Professional Excellence in Behavioral Health Real Estate Development 221

PART FOUR
PERMITTING, CONSTRUCTION & CLOSEOUT

15. Procurement and Preconstruction 237
16. Construction Management and Field Oversight 247
17. Construction Administration and Owner Engagement 259
18. Commissioning, Closeout, and Activation 269
19. Understanding California's Behavioral Health Transformation: The Behavioral Health Services Act (BHSA) and BHCIP, Behavioral Health Continuum Infrastructure Program 279

20. Licensing in Behavioral Health Real Estate 293
21. Call to Action for Behavioral Health Infrastructure 301

About the Author, BRIAN JONES 307
Glossary of Real Estate Development Terms 311
Resources for Behavioral Health Real Estate Development Support in California 319

WELCOME TO "THE WELLSPRING"

Welcome to "The Wellspring," your comprehensive professional guide for navigating the intricate landscape of behavioral health real estate development. This book serves as an essential deep resource, providing the insights, strategies, and hard-won wisdom necessary for executing infrastructure develoments that can and will transform lives and strengthen communities across California and beyond.

The Wellspring was written to empower professionals to create behavioral health facilities that are clinically sound, financially viable, and deeply responsive to the communities they serve. It's a guide for those who are ready to build not just faster—but smarter, more intentionally, and in ways that truly serve patients, providers, and the public good.

The metaphor matters.

A wellspring is a steady source of hidden and rising potential, bringing life and sustainability, if cultivated and used wisely. Good projects are the same. They draw on deep, reliable inputs: clinical insight, licensing knowledge, design that calms, financing that pencils, and community trust. When these sources converge, they cultivate successful humans & programs that last.

MISSION AND AUDIENCE

This manual serves owners, operators, public leaders, community stakeholders, and delivery teams in behavioral health. Use it to reduce risk, build winning teams, shorten schedules, and raise the quality of care environments. Every chapter turns principles into steps you can apply this week.

HOW TO USE THIS BOOK

Start at the beginning or start with the chapter that matches your next decision.

Engage your Owner's Advisor early to align design with licensing and funding.

Share the best practice bullets with your team to drive clarity.

Apply checklists and cross-checks before you commit to scope, schedule, or cost.

WHAT WE BELIEVE

"Dignity is non-negotiable in every space."

"Teamwork makes the Dream work."

"Early planning prevents most redesign and delay."

"Trauma-informed, biophilic design improves outcomes for patients and staff."

Great leadership enrolls others in a shared vision, constant clarity, and compassionate care.

With faith and gratitude,

Brian B. Jones
Founder & CEO, BHSME
www.bhsme.org

INTRODUCTION

The United States is facing an unprecedented behavioral health crisis -and with it, an urgent need for new facilities that can be planned, funded, and built faster, smarter, and with greater integrity. The Wellspring was written to meet that need.

Drawing on more than 25 years of real estate development experience and first-hand leadership of California's historic $5.5 billion Behavioral Health Continuum Infrastructure Program (BHCIP), this book provides a practical, battle-tested manual for healthcare leaders, counties, nonprofits, and developers. It bridges the gap between vision and execution, showing how to navigate complex funding, permitting, design, and construction with speed and confidence.

Inside, you'll find best practices, proven frameworks, and lessons learned from hundreds of behavioral health projects -distilled into clear strategies that any team can apply. From assembling the right experts, to avoiding costly delays, to ensuring regulatory compliance, The Wellspring equips you with the tools to deliver healing environments that restore dignity, strengthen communities, and change lives.

This book is designed to be your professional wellspring, a reliable source of guidance throughout every stage of development. Together we will explore the full life cycle of real estate development: from visioning and design, through permitting and construction, to licensing and operational readiness. Each chapter offers insights and best practices that support better decisions and foster the collaborative partnerships needed to transform ideas into reality.

This is not just a manual -it is a call to action. The time to build is now.

A NOTE FROM THE AUTHOR

> "Success is not the key to happiness. Happiness is the key to success. If you love what you are doing, you will be successful."
>
> ALBERT SCHWEITZER

Behavioral health is not a side issue. It is the heartbeat of our families, our communities, and our future. When care fails, lives unravel. When access lags, suffering deepens. Outdated buildings, long waitlists, and broken systems leave too many without hope. We cannot accept this. *The Wellspring* is both a guide and a promise—to show how we can build faster, smarter, and with compassion at the core.

I did not set out to write a book. I set out to help people I loved. Friends. Families. Neighbors. Real people facing real problems. Along the way, I discovered something sobering: even the best intentions collapse without strong foundations. Projects stall. Budgets explode. Teams misalign. Hope fades. But when clarity, purpose, and collaboration guide the process, results follow. Lives change. Communities heal. That is why this book exists.

My path into this work has been long and deeply personal. More than twenty years in real estate development taught me that buildings are never just walls and roofs.

They are vessels for human dignity. I've walked empty lots with providers who had nothing but a dream and a shoestring budget. I've sat with families desperate for care, waiting months for a space that did not yet exist. I've seen public officials struggle to balance urgent needs with limited resources. And I've stood beside builders, clinicians, and community leaders who refused to give up. These moments shaped me. They convinced me that when we bring people together around a shared mission, transformation happens.

That mission became BHSME.org, the practice I founded to help hospitals, counties, nonprofits, and developers deliver best-in-class behavioral health facilities. Our work is challenging, but it matters. Along the way I've drawn strength and guidance from professional communities that set the highest standards: the American Institute of Architects (AIA), the Design-Build Institute of America (DBIA), the Academy for Neuroscience for Architecture (ANFA), the California Department of Health Care Services (DHCS), the Department of Health Care Access and Information (HCAI), the Department of Social Services (DSS), and the California Department of Housing and Community Development (HCD). Their advocacy and leadership remind us that this healing work is not only urgent, but also possible.

The need is staggering. In California alone, hundreds of thousands of people struggle to access timely behavioral health treatment, while facilities lag decades behind demand. This gap is not just a statistic—it is the lived reality of families waiting for care, providers burning out, and communities breaking under the strain. It is also proof of why new approaches, rooted in speed, efficiency, and compassion, are essential.

This book is for everyone who shares in the responsibility to close that gap. For the nonprofit leader piecing together funding. For the county director navigating policy. For the developer building something new in a place that has waited too long. For the philanthropist seeking to give where it matters most. For the clinician, the housing agency, the policymaker. Whether you are starting small or leading on a statewide scale, my hope is that you will find tools here to move forward with clarity and confidence.

Because success in this field is not about one discipline—it is about people. Success happens when the right people gather early and often. When they listen first. When they build not just for speed, but for dignity. When design serves healing and recovery. When process honors compassion. When leadership holds integrity. Done well, this work touches not only patients but families, staff, and entire communities.

I do not have all the answers. None of us do. But I have seen what works. I have seen projects that seemed impossible come to life because the right team chose to lead with courage, creativity, and collaboration. That is why I wrote *The Wellspring*: to put those lessons, tools, and practices into your hands.

The name matters. A wellspring is a source. A beginning. Water that rises from deep within the earth, flowing fresh, steady, and true. It sustains life. It renews what is dry. In the same way, let this book be a source for you to draw inspiration, insight, and direction.

Together, we can do more than construct buildings. We can create places of renewal. We can restore hope. We can weave healing into the very foundations of our communities. This is the promise of *The Wellspring*—and it begins with you.

With gratitude,

Brian B. Jones

www.bhsme.org

PART ONE
SETTING THE VISION

Chapter 1

FOUNDATIONS of Behavioral Health Real Estate Development

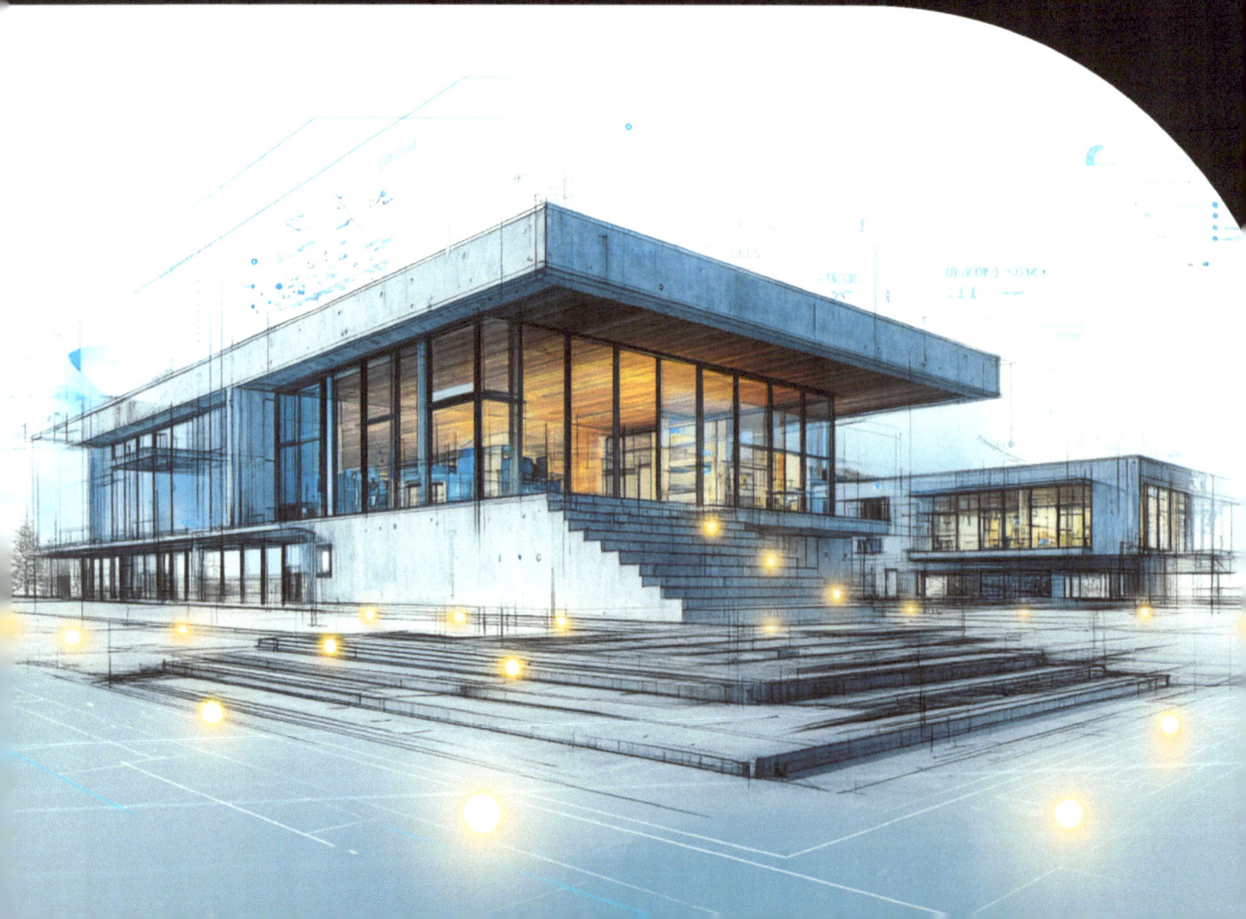

CHAPTER 1

FOUNDATIONS OF BEHAVIORAL HEALTH REAL ESTATE DEVELOPMENT

WHAT YOU WILL LEARN IN THIS CHAPTER

- **Real Estate Development Project Success Factors**
- **The Urgent Demand for Behavioral Health Facilities**
- **Unique Complexities of Behavioral Health Care Environments**
- **Licensing, Care Models, and Regulatory Priorities**
- **Timelines, Funding Cycles, and Delivery Constraints**
- **Defining Mission, Values, and Measurable Goals**

Definiteness of purpose turns an inspiring mission into measurable, staged outcomes. In behavioral health real estate, that means naming exactly who you serve, what opens when, and how each phase reduces risk while protecting dignity. Clarity concentrates effort. In complex, regulated delivery, it also aligns teams and shortens debate. Define the end state, then translate vision into phase-gated milestones the entire team can see and move toward together.

Convert aspiration into scope, schedule, and budget that withstand public scrutiny and clinical needs. Tie purpose to California funding cycles, licensing windows, and community expectations so work advances when the window opens. The Owner's Advisor reinforces this with a master decision log, weekly dashboards, and a steady review rhythm that turns direction into visible progress. Purpose becomes performance when every choice maps back to the aim. If operating outside California, map this to your state authority and funding calendar.

DEFINITENESS OF PURPOSE: FROM MISSION TO MILESTONES

Why it matters

Definiteness of purpose turns an inspiring mission into **measurable, staged outcomes**. In behavioral health real estate, it means stating **who you serve, what opens when**, and **how each phase reduces risk while protecting dignity**.

1. Define the End State
    - **Population & services:** Name exactly **who** you serve and **which programs** you will operate.
    - **Operational outcomes:** Specify target capacity, access metrics, quality and safety goals.
    - **Facility end state:** Describe the fully built environment you're moving toward.
2. Phase-Gate the Path
    - **What opens when:** Sequence activation (e.g., crisis stabilization → outpatient → residential).
    - **Risk reduction:** Show how each phase **de-risks** financing, licensing, staffing, and operations.
    - **Visibility:** Publish a **phase-gated milestone map** the entire team can see and track.
3. Convert Vision into Scope, Schedule, Budget
    - **Scope:** Translate aspiration into **program, rooms, systems, and performance criteria**.
    - **Schedule:** Build a **realistic timeline** with decision gates and inspection/licensing holds.
    - **Budget:** Tie scope to a **defensible pro forma** that stands up to public and clinical scrutiny.

4. Align to External Calendars
   - **California focus:** Sync to **funding cycles, licensing windows,** and **community expectations** so work advances when the window opens.
   - **Other states:** Map the same logic to your **state authority and funding calendar**.
5. Make Purpose Operable (Owner's Advisor)
   - **Master decision log** capturing commitments, owners, and due dates.
   - **Weekly dashboards** for schedule, budget, risks, and readiness.
   - **Review cadence** (phase gates, design milestones, pre-licensing checks) that turns direction into **visible progress**.

RULE OF ALIGNMENT

Purpose → Plan → Proof. Every choice maps back to the aim. If it doesn't, **reframe or remove it**.

QUICK CHECKLIST

☐ End state defined (population, programs, capacity, outcomes)
☐ Phase-gated milestones published and tracked
☐ Scope/Schedule/Budget integrated and defensible
☐ Calendars aligned (funding, licensing, community)
☐ OA tools live: decision log, dashboards, review rhythm

REAL ESTATE DEVELOPMENT PROJECT SUCCESS FACTORS

What makes a behavioral health real estate project succeed?

Success is set at the outset. The strongest projects intentionally integrate the strategies below to stay on **budget, scope, and schedule** while delivering clinical impact.

A) COMPREHENSIVE PLANNING & VISION

Ground decisions in a long-view strategy informed by data and community voice. Plan for:

- **Population needs & service gaps**
- **Program & treatment modalities**
- **Future scalability & adaptability**

B) STRONG LEADERSHIP & INTERDISCIPLINARY COLLABORATION

Build a team-driven approach that unites:

- **Healthcare-savvy developers** to guide delivery and anticipate challenges
- **Behavioral health professionals** to shape function and care flows
- **Policy/funding experts** to navigate regulations and capital sources

C) FINANCIAL SUSTAINABILITY & BUDGET DISCIPLINE

Design for viability through:

- **Diverse funding streams** to reduce risk
- **Operational efficiency models** aligned to reimbursement
- **Proactive risk management** to prevent overruns

D) COMMUNITY INTEGRATION & PUBLIC SUPPORT

Treat the facility as a **community asset**:

- **Engage stakeholders early & often**
- **Design inside/out to invite participation** (wellness/shared program spaces)

- **Adopt policies** that demonstrate long-term commitment to local well-being

E) NEUROLOGICALLY ATTUNED FACILITY DESIGN → BETTER OUTCOMES

Evolve beyond containment to **healing-centered design**:

- **Therapeutic environments** (mind–body–spirit) → nervous system coherence
- **Privacy & dignity by design** → calmer, safer experiences
- **Holistic wellness integration** (nutrition, fitness, community) → whole-person care

> "We shape our buildings, and afterwards our buildings shape us."
>
> WINSTON CHURCHILL

UNDERSTANDING THE URGENT DEMAND FOR BEHAVIORAL HEALTH FACILITIES

Across the U.S.—and acutely in **California**—mental health and substance use needs are at historic highs. Infrastructure has not kept pace, leaving people underserved and communities strained. Behavioral health real estate is now a **public health necessity**, not a niche.

A behavioral health facility is not just a container for services—it is **part of the therapy**. **Location, access, design, and functionality** can spell the difference between recovery and a missed opportunity. Done well, these become **sanctuaries for healing**, engines of community health, and durable public assets.

California can lead again—pairing innovation with equity—to deliver environments that **protect dignity, empower recovery, and meet urgent need with precision**.

> "Design is not just what it looks like and feels like. **Design is how it works.**"
>
> STEVE JOBS

UNIQUE COMPLEXITIES OF BEHAVIORAL HEALTH CARE ENVIRONMENTS

Designing and developing behavioral health facilities requires navigating **clinical demands, community dynamics, financing structures, and regulatory frameworks.** Unlike general healthcare or residential projects, behavioral health environments must balance **psychological sensitivity, physical safety, and clinical effectiveness.**

CORE COMPLEXITIES

Needs Assessments

- Use **local data and provider input** to define the most urgent services (residential treatment, detox, crisis stabilization, etc.).

Design for Trauma-Informed Care

- Promote **safety, calm, and autonomy** through evidence-based design: natural light, biophilic elements, low-stimulation zones, and clear sightlines.

Workforce Realities

- Address clinician shortages and burnout with **staff support spaces, operational efficiency, and telehealth infrastructure.**

Community Resistance (NIMBY)

- Mitigate opposition with **early outreach, public education, and trusted partnerships** to position the facility as a community asset.

NAVIGATING LICENSING, CARE MODELS, AND REGULATIONS

Behavioral health projects operate within **dense regulatory frameworks** that must be anticipated and integrated from the outset.

KEY REGULATORY CONCERNS

- **Licensing Requirements**: Different facility types (outpatient, residential, detox) require distinct state licensure with strict physical plant criteria.
- **Care Model Integration**: Layouts must support therapeutic modalities (integrated care, trauma-informed models, co-occurring disorders treatment).
- **Building Code Compliance**: Ensure alignment with **ADA, Title 24, HCAI/OSHPD standards, ligature resistance, and infection control.**
- **Agency Engagement**: Proactively coordinate with **DHCS, HCAI (formerly OSHPD), Fire Marshal, and local planning boards** to prevent approval delays.

Failure to embed these priorities early risks redesigns, costly delays, or even non-licensable facilities.

TIMELINES, FUNDING CYCLES, AND DELIVERY CONSTRAINTS

Behavioral health projects face a paradox: **urgent demand vs. complex delivery.** Success requires balancing speed with quality and compliance.

Challenges

- **Funding Complexity**: Blend of Medi-Cal reimbursements, MHSA grants, local housing funds, and private capital -each with unique cycles.
- **Schedule Synchronization**: Align entitlements, grants, procurement, and design milestones to maintain momentum.
- **Permitting and Approvals**: Engage early with regulators and communities to **avoid bottlenecks.**
- **Construction Strategy**: Leverage **modular methods, phased occupancy, and CM-at-Risk contracts** for speed and cost control.

Key Insight: Agility is as critical as planning. Teams must adapt quickly to shifting **policies, construction delays, or funding windows** while safeguarding clinical outcomes.

MISSION, VISION, AND VALUES

> "Plans are nothing; planning is everything."
>
> DWIGHT D. EISENHOWER

Strategic behavioral health real estate begins with **mission clarity** and **shared values.**

Foundational Elements

- **Community-Driven Visioning**: Rooted in **local context, public health trends, and service gaps.**
- **Measurable Success Criteria**: Define **clinical outcomes, utilization targets, and quality metrics** from day one.
- **Stakeholder Alignment**: Foster cross-sector partnerships -providers, funders, policymakers, architects, and neighbors.

- **Cultural Competency**: Ensure facilities resonate with the populations served through **design, staffing, and programming.**

When rooted in these principles, facilities transcend construction and become **long-term engines of healing and transformation.**

KEY CONSIDERATIONS IN BEHAVIORAL HEALTH REAL ESTATE DEVELOPMENT

The **cornerstones of successful project delivery** in this demanding sector:

1. Needs Assessment & Market Demand
2. Strategic Site Selection
3. Healing-Centered Design
4. Compliance-Driven Planning
5. Financial Sustainability
6. Community Engagement
7. Operational Readiness

Summary: Success in behavioral health facility development lies in **balancing urgency with precision, community with compliance, and vision with execution.**

WHAT MAKES A PROJECT WORK

Every successful behavioral health facility rests on a few essential principles.

1. **Plan Across Disciplines**
    - Use **real data** to define needs.
    - Develop a **long-term budget** covering both construction and operations.
    - Prepare early for **licensing and compliance** requirements.

2. **Involve the Community**
   - **Listen first**: communities are partners, not just stakeholders.
   - Be **open and transparent** from the outset.
   - Collaborate with **local leaders** who already have community trust.
3. **Design for Healing & Flexibility**
   - Create environments that are **safe, open, and calming**.
   - Ensure designs can **adapt as care models evolve**.
   - Integrate **sustainability and energy efficiency** from day one.
4. **Moving Forward Together**
   - No single group can solve the behavioral health crisis. Progress requires governments, healthcare leaders, developers, and communities working as one.
5. **Align Funding & Policy**
   - Strengthen programs like **Medi-Cal** and **CalAIM**.
   - **Simplify approval processes** for facilities.
   - Provide **incentives** for developers who build healing spaces.
6. **Stay Open to Innovation**
   - Plan facilities with **future care models** in mind: telehealth, mobile crisis teams, digital tools.
   - Use **data and technology** to improve both care delivery and operations.

Summary: Projects work best when they are **planned holistically, rooted in community, designed for healing, and supported by aligned policy and innovation.**

FRONT LINE STORY #1. "OVERCOMING CHALLENGES: NAVIGATING REGULATORY HURDLES IN PSYCHIATRIC HOSPITAL DEVELOPMENT"

> "Opportunities don't happen. You create them."
>
> CHRIS GROSSER, REAL ESTATE DEVELOPER

“FRONT LINE STORY #1” I want to start here with my first of 33 personal "front line stories" because this experience clearly illustrates the many challenges we face in behavioral health development.

Acute psychiatric hospitals require specialized design elements, such as ligature-resistant fixtures, secure environments, and various program rooms. All of these demand significant resources and expertise. Unfortunately, the initial pricing failed to reflect these complexities, leaving the ownership group with a budget underestimated by more than 50 percent.

Upon realizing the magnitude of the oversight, the ownership group scrambled to assemble a new design-build team with healthcare expertise. We undertook a redesign that reduced the building from 28,000 sf to 20,000 sf, bringing the budget down to $32 million. The process involved rigorous value engineering and strategic tenant improvements. Our team aligned priorities around cost containment and stakeholder coordination, ensuring everyone understood the necessary scope adjustments.

This experience reinforced the critical importance of early collaboration and effective communication in project management. Navigating the challenges of this project highlighted the necessity of expertise and thorough planning in our industry. By prioritizing strategic decision-making, we can better manage risks and deliver facilities that meet the critical needs of the communities we serve.

THE POWER OF TEAMWORK IN REAL ESTATE DEVELOPMENT

Real estate development is a **complex, multidisciplinary process** that demands seamless coordination. Delivering behavioral health facilities **on budget, on scope, and on schedule** depends on teamwork -bringing together top professionals into a **cohesive, high-performing team.**

BEST PRACTICE PRINCIPLES

1. **Teamwork as the Foundation of Excellence**
   - Excellence requires the **collaboration of diverse professionals** working as one.
2. **The Owner's Advisor as Team Integrator**
   - The Owner's Advisor ensures each expert stays **aligned with the project mission** and goals.
3. **Aligning Mission, Vision, and Values**
   - A unified vision creates **cohesion, efficiency, and purpose-driven execution.**
4. **Collaborative Scope Definition**
   - Early collaboration among **architects, engineers, compliance managers, and financial managers** prevents costly redesigns and delays.
5. **Interdisciplinary Schedule Management**
   - Guided by **expediters and construction managers,** collaborative scheduling anticipates dependencies and mitigates delays.
6. **Budgeting & Financial Oversight as a Team Effort**
   - When **financial managers, brokers, and contractors** work together, cost overruns are minimized.
7. **Team-Wide Quality Assurance**
   - A culture of **excellence across all disciplines** ensures safe, effective, and durable facilities.
8. **Unified Stakeholder Engagement**
   - **Community relations and legal counsel** help align communities, agencies, and investors, preventing opposition and facilitating integration.
9. **Collective Risk Management**
   - **Compliance managers, urban planners, and technology specialists** collaborate to create resilient, adaptable projects.

10. **Continuous Learning Mindset**
    - Teams that share knowledge and feedback remain **adaptive, innovative, and future-ready.**
11. **Celebrating Success and Contributions**
    - Recognizing and celebrating achievements boosts **morale, cohesion, and long-term performance.**

✅ SUMMARY:

Teamwork is not just a soft skill -it is the **structural framework** that ensures behavioral health real estate projects are delivered with **precision, resilience, and impact.**

TYPE 2 FUN: "TIMELESS MISSION, VISION & VALUES: FOUNDATIONS OF MY WORK"

> "Real estate is an imperishable asset, ever increasing in value. It is the most solid security that human ingenuity has devised."
>
> RUSSELL SAGE, FINANCIER

At the core of our work in behavioral health and real estate development are the mission, vision, and values that guide our best practices and principles approach. These principles are deeply personal and stem from a lifelong exploration of the human experience, enriched by my academic background in Comparative Philosophy of Religion and an M.A. in Personality Psychology from Stanford. Such studies provide profound insights into wisdom traditions (from Zen Buddhism to Christian compassion) and modern science, including neuroscience and the concept of "type 2 fun." If you're unfamiliar with "type 2 fun," I encourage you to explore it. Its impact on our nervous system and the ever-evolving genetic sequencing of our DNA in each cell is remarkably positive. Successful type 2 fun experiences may soon prove to be key to rewiring our nervous system, overcoming behavioral health challenges, and restructuring our mental frameworks for resilience, balance, and excellence.

My core values are reflected in healthy and safe type 2 fun, including outdoor adventure, compassion, integrity, collaboration, and excellence. My professional and personal mission is to foster environments and consciousness that promote healing, growth, and connection. My vision is to cultivate a world where these values are at the forefront, creating communities that thrive through a shared purpose.

Over 30 years of international travels across Asia, India, Australia, Europe, and South, Central, and North America deepened my appreciation for architecture, sacred spaces, and collective community synergy, much like a natural harmony of earthly ecosystems. Professional and personal excellence demand a team committed to shared values, virtues, and vision. Misalignment is costly; clear communication, follow-through, and authenticity are non-negotiable. Ultimately, it is our shared humanity, and our commitment to love and truth, that lays the foundation for transformative work.

> "The greatest wealth is health."
>
> VIRGIL

LAYING THE GROUNDWORK FOR LASTING IMPACT

Behavioral health real estate development stands at the **intersection of urgency and opportunity.** With the growing mental health crisis, the demand for specialized healing environments is no longer aspirational -it is **foundational to community well-being and public health infrastructure.**

These projects are not typical real estate ventures. They require a rare **fusion of vision, expertise, compassion, and discipline** to succeed.

This chapter has laid out the **cornerstone principles of success**:

- Strategic planning
- Regulatory fluency
- Healing-centered design
- Financial discipline
- Community alignment

These elements form the **DNA of a well-executed behavioral health facility.** More than any checklist or codebook, what differentiates transformative projects is the **intentionality** behind every decision and the **values embedded** in every square foot of space.

BEST PRACTICES FOR A STRONG FOUNDATION

1. **Mission-Driven Vision**
   - Anchor the project in clear values and measurable outcomes that reflect the needs of real people, not just funding priorities.
2. **Early & Continuous Collaboration**
   - Engage behavioral health professionals, funders, developers, regulators, and community members throughout the process.
3. **Plan for Flexibility**
   - Design environments that are scalable, adaptable, and resilient to shifts in care models, technology, and demographics.
4. **Design for Dignity**
   - Incorporate natural light, privacy, biophilic design, and calming elements to foster spaces that support healing and recovery.

RISK MITIGATION STRATEGIES

- **Regulatory Complexity**: Engage licensing bodies (DHCS, HCAI/OSHPD) during pre-development to align requirements with facility planning.
- **Community Resistance**: Use transparent engagement campaigns to build trust, dispel stigma, and highlight public benefit.

- **Funding Gaps & Delays**: Layer capital stacks, build financial contingencies, and allow flexibility for grant cycles and reimbursements.
- **Operational Mismatch**: Collaborate with operators and clinicians to ensure design supports workflows and staffing realities.
- **Timeline Disruptions**: Adopt delivery models like CM-at-Risk or Progressive Design-Build to accelerate while maintaining accountability.

THE REAL ESTATE DEVELOPMENT PROCESS

Behavioral health real estate development is **structured, multifaceted, and disciplined.** A successful cycle typically unfolds over **2–3 years** and follows **six major phases:**

1. **Concept Planning**
2. **Due Diligence & Feasibility Analysis**
3. **Schematic Planning, Entitlements & Approvals**
4. **Construction Drawings & Permitting**
5. **General Contractor Evaluation & Contracting**
6. **Construction & Move-In**

WHY STRATEGIC PLANNING MATTERS

Strategic planning in behavioral health real estate is not a formality -it is the **foundation of success.**

- It ensures alignment of **scope, schedule, and budget** at every step.
- It integrates **financial, clinical, and regulatory perspectives.**
- It prevents missteps that lead to **delays, overruns, or non-licensable facilities.**

CORE TEAM FOR EACH PHASE

Each development phase builds upon the last and requires **seamless collaboration** among:

- Developers & Owners
- **Owner's Advisors**
- Architects & Engineers
- Construction Managers
- Financial Analysts
- Utility & Environmental Consultants

SUMMARY:

Every successful behavioral health facility begins with a **clear vision** and is carried forward by a **disciplined process.** Intentionality, foresight, and collaboration transform facilities from buildings into **healing environments** with lasting community impact.

6 PHASES OF REAL ESTATE DEVELOPMENT

Behavioral health real estate projects typically span **24–48 months** and progress through six critical phases. Each phase carries unique workflows, roles, challenges, and opportunities that move the project from **vision to successful operation.**

PHASE 1: CONCEPT PLANNING

- Define **vision, target population, and service model**
- Conduct **early market scans and site screenings**
- Develop a **preliminary development and operating budget**
- **Role of the Owner's Advisor:** Align stakeholders, unify direction, and establish expectations. This phase sets the tone for the entire project.

PHASE 2: DUE DILIGENCE & FEASIBILITY

- Environmental site assessments (**Phase I/II ESAs**)
- **Zoning and land use** verification
- **Dry utility coordination** and "will-serve" letters
- **Soil and geotechnical investigations**
- Creation of a **risk matrix and feasibility scoring model**

PHASE 3: SCHEMATIC DESIGN & ENTITLEMENTS

- **Schematic plans** and engineering coordination
- **CUP (Conditional Use Permit), CEQA, and environmental review**
- **Community engagement** and public hearings
- Budget adjustments based on entitlement outcomes

PHASE 4: CONSTRUCTION DRAWINGS & PERMITS

- Completion of **full Construction Document (CD) set** and agency submittals
- **Constructability reviews** and value engineering
- **Permit expediting and resubmittals** to resolve comments

PHASE 5: GENERAL CONTRACTOR SELECTION & CONTRACTING

- Issue **RFP, conduct interviews, and level bids**
- Negotiate **Guaranteed Maximum Price (GMP) or fixed-price contract**
- Finalize **schedule, budget, and key milestones**

PHASE 6: CONSTRUCTION & OCCUPANCY

- **Site mobilization** and field inspections
- Ongoing **quality assurance** and compliance oversight
- **Cost tracking** and monthly pay applications
- **Punch list completion, commissioning, and closeout**
- Achievement of **Certificate of Occupancy** and transition to operations

✅ SUMMARY:

These six phases form the **blueprint for successful behavioral health real estate development.** From concept through occupancy, each stage demands **precision, coordination, and proactive risk management** to ensure facilities are delivered **on time, on budget, and aligned with clinical and community needs.**

IN CONCLUSION: THOUGHT LEADERSHIP & A CALL TO BUILD BOLDLY AND RESPONSIBLY

At its core, behavioral health real estate is about more than square footage or licensing checklists; it's about hope. It's about creating spaces where individuals at their most vulnerable can rediscover their strength. It's about investing in environments that not only house care, but elevate it. And it's about building in ways that reflect the dignity, diversity, and humanity of those we serve.

The role of the Owner's Advisor and development team is to be more than builders. We must be stewards of recovery, catalysts for equity, and architects of transformation.

As we look forward, we must reframe these projects not as liabilities to manage but as investments in long-term public health and social infrastructure. By building on a foundation of best practices, strategic foresight, and deeply human-centered design, we can deliver facilities that don't just open their doors; they open the path to healing, resilience, and lasting impact.

Let us build not only for today's needs but for tomorrow's recovery.

> "There is no power for change greater than a community discovering what it cares about."
>
> MARGARET J. WHEATLEY

Chapter 2

Strategic Planning and **FEASABILITY** Analysis

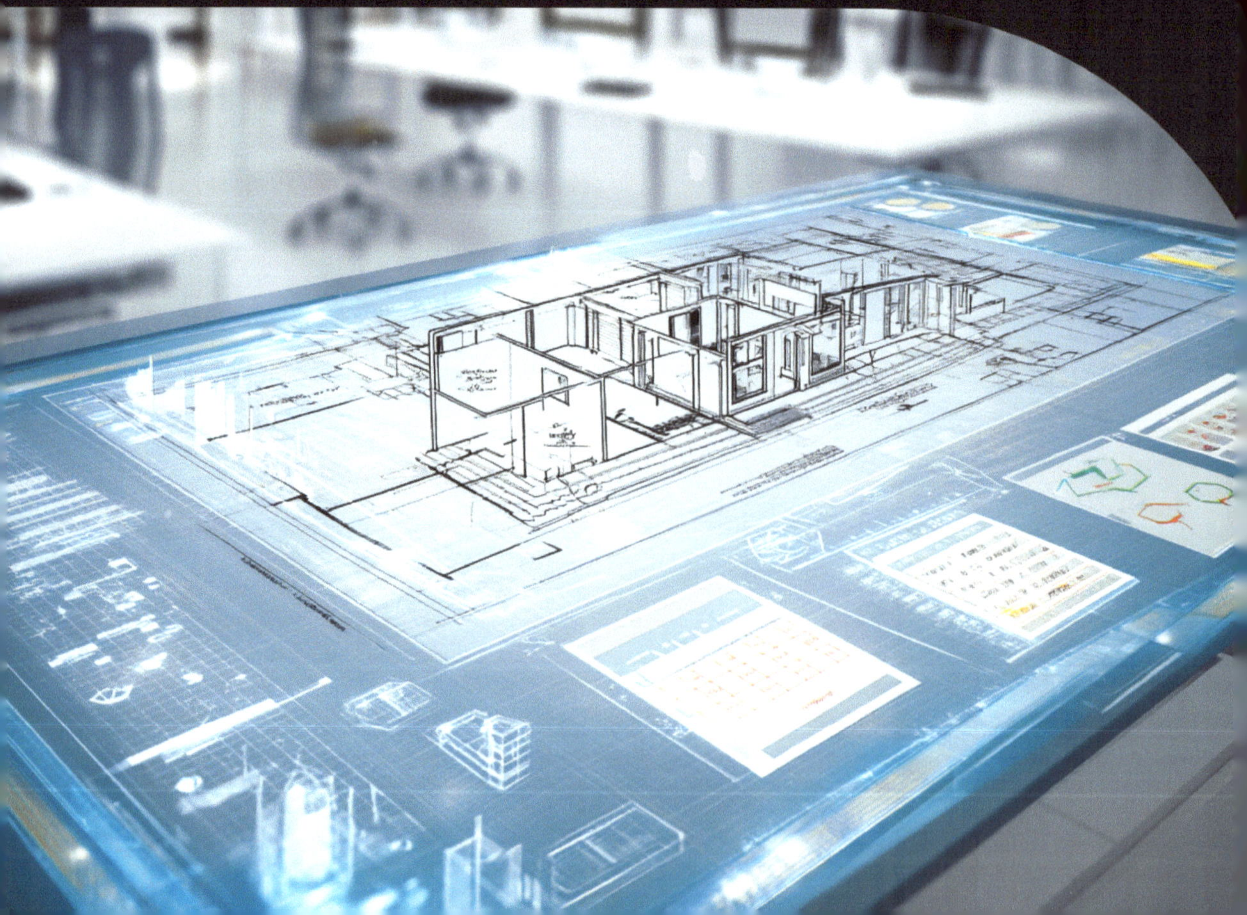

CHAPTER 2
STRATEGIC PLANNING AND FEASIBILITY ANALYSIS

WHAT YOU WILL LEARN IN THIS CHAPTER

This chapter provides a structured foundation for behavioral health real estate development. Readers will gain practical insights and applied strategies across seven critical areas:

1. Market Studies & Needs Assessments

Learn how to evaluate demand, identify service gaps, and align facility planning with actual community and clinical needs.

2. Site Selection Criteria for Behavioral Health

Understand the unique requirements for location, including safety, accessibility, visibility, and proximity to healthcare and transit services.

3. Zoning, Access, & Neighborhood Integration

Explore how zoning laws, entitlement processes, and community dynamics shape site viability and long-term acceptance.

4. Preliminary Budgeting & Pro Forma Modeling

Build accurate development and operating budgets that integrate financing, grant cycles, and reimbursement streams.

5. Risk Identification & Mitigation Strategies

Anticipate financial, regulatory, and operational risks early to prevent costly delays and redesigns.

6. Due Diligence Process

Review the technical, legal, and environmental steps necessary to validate project feasibility before acquisition or development.

7. Real Estate Development Process

Gain a roadmap of the full development cycle -from concept to occupancy -highlighting workflows, timelines, and best practices.

Organized planning is how leaders turn good intentions into reliable outcomes. Define decision gates, map critical dependencies, and assign single-threaded owners for material risks. Plans organize both thought and effort, creating shared clarity that reduces rework and accelerates delivery. In this phase, discipline beats improvisation, and evidence beats opinion.

Build a planning system that holds under pressure. Maintain a living risk register, a milestone roadmap synced to funding windows, and a weekly forum where facts outrank assumptions. In California, integrate licensing constraints, entitlement timelines, and capital stack realities so the plan is credible on paper and resilient in the field. The result is a team that knows what happens next and why it matters. If operating outside California, map this to your state authority and funding calendar.

Strategic planning is the bedrock of successful behavioral health real estate development. While construction milestones and design innovation often steal the spotlight, it is the thoughtful, data-informed groundwork laid in the early phases that determines whether a project thrives, stalls, or fails. In this chapter, we explore the foundational elements of planning and feasibility that ensure projects are aligned with real-world needs, financially viable, and ready to navigate a complex regulatory and community landscape.

FRONT LINE STORY #2. THE RIGHT SIZE FOR SUCCESS

I remember one of the most pivotal moments in my career as an Owner's Advisor. I was brought into a project that, on paper, looked ambitious and inspiring: a 180-bed Substance Use Disorder (SUD) treatment facility that was intended to be the flagship of a new behavioral health campus. The sponsor had passion, funding interest, and a big vision. But as I began walking through the seven steps of feasibility—market study, site selection, zoning, budgeting, risk review, due diligence, and process mapping—it became clear that the project was not right-sized for reality.

The market analysis was my first warning sign. Community need was real, but the payer mix and referral streams could not sustain 180 beds. Staffing projections showed the same problem: in California's strained healthcare workforce, simply finding enough licensed clinicians, nurses, and support staff would be an insurmountable challenge. As we ran preliminary pro formas, the construction budget ballooned, the operating costs escalated, and the business model bent under the weight of assumptions that looked inspiring in a slide deck but fragile in practice.

I had to bring the leadership team back to first principles: evidence beats opinion. What did the community actually need? What could the organization actually staff, fund, and sustain without overreaching? That's when we began the disciplined process of right-sizing.

Through zoning review and site analysis, we identified a portion of the property that could accommodate a smaller footprint. We modeled a reduced scope—24 beds instead of 180—and re-ran the numbers. The construction budget fell dramatically, operating costs aligned with realistic reimbursement streams, staffing became attainable, and the regulatory hurdles became far more manageable.

Was it a hard conversation? Absolutely. Scaling down a grand vision to something more modest always feels, at first, like a step backward. But the truth is, it was a step toward sustainability. The smaller facility meant the sponsor could actually open, operate, and succeed without risking organizational collapse. The revised plan created breathing room for growth, rather than immediate pressure to perform at a scale that would likely have led to failure.

That project became a lasting lesson for me: right-sizing is not a compromise—it's a strategy. It is the difference between building something impressive that never survives its own weight, versus building something achievable that grows into a stable platform for future expansion. In the end, the 24-bed project not only got built, it thrived. And the organization gained the confidence, credibility, and cash flow to consider future growth at the right pace, on their own terms.

Every time I sit with a sponsor now, I remind them: the foundation of success in behavioral health real estate development is not about building the biggest project. It's about building the right project—aligned with need, budget, staffing, and mission. That's the discipline of feasibility, and that's what turns good intentions into reliable outcomes.

MARKET STUDIES & NEEDS ASSESSMENTS

> "Without data, you're just another person with an opinion."
>
> W. EDWARDS DEMING

A successful behavioral health real estate project starts with a **clear, data-driven picture of community demand**. Market research and needs assessments turn intentions into **actionable, locally grounded plans**.

WHAT MARKET STUDIES MEASURE

- **Prevalence** of behavioral health conditions
- **Service utilization** (hospitals, corrections, outpatient)
- **Demographics** (age, race, income, insurance status)

- **Provider capacity & waitlists**
- **Policy context** (state/local funding initiatives, delivery reforms)

Outcome: Inputs for investment decisions, regulatory filings, and architectural programming.

COMMUNITY-FOCUSED NEEDS ASSESSMENTS

Qualitative complements that capture lived experience:

- **Focus groups & interviews** with leaders and service users
- **Public health data** (MHSA plans, CHNAs, local health agencies)
- **Access barriers** (language, transportation, stigma, cultural fit)
- **High-need populations** (justice-involved, TAY, veterans)

Outcome: Ensures solutions are **clinically relevant** and **socially responsive**.

KEY DATA SOURCES

- SAMHSA **Behavioral Health Barometers**
- **County Health Rankings**
- **Medi-Cal/CalAIM** datasets
- **OSHPD/HCAI** hospital discharge data
- **U.S. Census / ACS**
- Local **MHSA Innovation Plans**

SITE SELECTION CRITERIA SPECIFIC TO BEHAVIORAL HEALTH

> "Real estate is not just about buildings. It's about access, context, and community."
>
> BRIAN JONES

Site choice is a **clinical and operational decision** with long-term implications.

CRITICAL SELECTION CRITERIA

- **Transit & services proximity** (care, housing, social supports)
- **Distance from triggering environments** / high-crime areas
- **Zoning compatibility** and **community acceptance**
- **Patient privacy + therapeutic outdoor spaces**
- **Infrastructure readiness** (utilities, broadband, fire access)

Tip: Use a **weighted evaluation matrix** with input from clinicians, neighbors, and public agencies.

COMMON RED FLAGS

- **Environmental contamination** (brownfields)
- **Unfavorable zoning** with low political support for variances
- **High neighborhood resistance (NIMBY)**
- **Weak infrastructure** (septic limits, poor broadband, aging utilities)

ZONING, ACCESS TO SERVICES & NEIGHBORHOOD INTEGRATION

> "Planning is bringing the future into the present so you can do something about it now."
>
> ALAN LAKEIN

Zoning/entitlements are a leading cause of project delays—plan early and engage broadly.

ZONING & ENTITLEMENTS

- Conduct **early zoning analysis** to confirm viability and avoid deal-breakers
- Anticipate **CUPs** for mental health uses; know local processes (hearings, CEQA/NEPA)
- Engage **zoning attorneys & planners** early; start **public outreach before** submitting

NEIGHBORHOOD INTEGRATION STRATEGIES

- **Contextual design:** Align architecture/landscape with local character
- **Shared community spaces** for wellness and education
- **Community advisory boards** for post-occupancy dialogue and accountability
- **Public milestones:** Groundbreakings/ribbon cuttings to build goodwill

FRONT LINE STORY #3. MARKET ANALYSIS INSIGHT: UNCOVERING HIDDEN NEEDS

Our team was deep into a feasibility study for a new adult crisis stabilization unit (CSU). The county's official health plan pointed to a clear need, the funding seemed aligned, and all our preliminary work supported this direction. But something felt incomplete. The data we were using, while official, was nearly two years old, a lifetime in the world of public health.

Driven by a hunch, I started digging deeper, pulling raw data from local hospital emergency departments, school districts, and pediatricians. A startling pattern emerged: a dramatic threefold increase in emergency psychiatric visits for adolescents over the past 18 months. This was a silent crisis, a wave of need that was building so fast it hadn't yet been reflected in the county's formal strategic plans. The system was focused on adults, but the most urgent, unaddressed need was for youth.

I brought the findings to our stakeholders. Pivoting the project was a significant risk. It meant re-evaluating our financial model, our architectural program, and our operational plan. But the data was undeniable. We made the call to shift our focus to an adolescent CSU. It was a challenging, complex pivot that required re-engaging our partners and making the case for a project that wasn't on anyone's official roadmap. Six months later, the county declared a pediatric mental health state of emergency, and our project was suddenly at the forefront of the solution. It was a powerful lesson in how market analysis is not just about confirming what we already know, but about uncovering the needs that no one is seeing yet.

> "Without strategy, execution is aimless. Without execution, strategy is useless."
>
> MORRIS CHANG

PRELIMINARY BUDGETING & PRO FORMA MODELING

> "A budget is telling your money where to go instead of wondering where it went."
>
> DAVE RAMSEY

A sound financial model is both **map and mirror**—it charts the path and reflects assumptions that demand scrutiny and discipline.

DEVELOPMENT BUDGET COMPONENTS

- **Land**: acquisition, due diligence, holding costs
- **Soft Costs**: legal, architectural/engineering, permitting, environmental reviews
- **Hard Costs**: construction, site work, **FF&E**, contingencies
- **Financing**: interest reserve, lender fees, closing costs

- **Operational Reserve**: cash buffer for early stabilization

PRO FORMA MODELING — WHAT TO INCLUDE

- **Revenue by service line**: Medi-Cal, private pay, grants, contracts
- **Operating expenses**: tied to staffing ratios, acuity levels, and hours of operation
- **Capital metrics: DSCR, IRR, NPV**
- **Sensitivity analyses**: reimbursement rate shifts, census shortfalls, schedule slippage
- **Collaboration**: build the model with finance consultants **and** provider leadership; incorporate input from local funders/authorities

RISK IDENTIFICATION & MITIGATION STRATEGIES

> "In preparing for battle, I have always found that plans are useless, but planning is indispensable."
>
> DWIGHT D. EISENHOWER

The #1 reason behavioral health facilities fail to launch is **unmanaged risk**. Plan rigorously—and realistically—for what can go wrong.

KEY RISK AREAS

- **Entitlement/zoning denial**
- **Cost escalation** beyond contingencies
- **Licensing or accreditation failure**
- **Insufficient operating cash** post-construction
- **Community resistance** and political backlash

RISK MANAGEMENT FRAMEWORK

- **Contingencies**: budget, schedule, and scope buffers
- **Insurance & bonding**: builder's risk, E&O, general liability
- **Legal structures**: MOUs, JV agreements, clear responsibilities
- **Fallbacks**: alternative sites, **phased delivery** options
- **Scenario planning**: best/base/worst-case forecasts with trigger actions

QUICK CHECKLIST

☐ Complete development budget (land → reserves)
☐ Pro forma with DSCR/IRR/NPV and sensitivities
☐ Funding & reimbursement assumptions validated with payors/funders
☐ Risk register with owners, mitigations, and review cadence
☐ Contingency levels set and protected (no early erosion)

THE CRITICAL ROLE OF DUE DILIGENCE IN BEHAVIORAL HEALTH REAL ESTATE DEVELOPMENT

In behavioral health real estate, the due diligence process is not a formality -it is a **high-stakes, multi-disciplinary investigation** that determines a project's viability, cost, safety, compliance, and timeline. Whether for ground-up construction or rehabilitation of an existing facility, due diligence is the foundation of sustainable, compliant, and successful development.

Projects that skip or shortcut due diligence routinely face:

- Cost overruns
- Failed permitting
- Environmental liabilities
- Missed timelines
- Unbuildable conditions

Given the **specialized regulations, safety standards, and funding cycles** tied to behavioral health, inadequate due diligence can be fatal to project success.

This section outlines **best practices across technical, legal, financial, and regulatory due diligence.**

I. SITE & LEGAL DUE DILIGENCE

1. Title Report & Legal Review

- Order preliminary title report from a licensed title company.
- Examine for:
  - Easements, liens, CC&Rs, reversion clauses, or restrictions.
  - Shared access agreements, utilities, or reciprocal easements.
- Confirm rights for behavioral healthcare uses ("residential," "outpatient," "crisis," etc.).
- Engage real estate counsel to validate zoning entitlements and contract rights.

2. Zoning & Entitlement Analysis

- Verify current zoning and allowable land uses.
- Request Zoning Verification Letter from municipality.
- Determine requirements for:
  - CUPs or variances.
  - Density, height, FAR, and parking.
- Ensure General Plan consistency.
- Identify restrictions that could block behavioral health occupancy.

3. ALTA/NSPS Land Title Survey

- Commission full survey to:
  - Locate boundaries, easements, encroachments, setbacks.
  - Overlay with title report for consistency.

    - Identify flood zones, topography, adjacent parcel context, and access points.

II. ENVIRONMENTAL & PHYSICAL DUE DILIGENCE

1. Phase I & II Environmental Site Assessments (ESA)

- **Phase I ESA (ASTM E1527-21):** Review historical land use, hazardous materials, prior activity, and interview owners.
- **Phase II ESA (if needed):** Test soil, groundwater, and vapor; estimate remediation feasibility and costs.

2. Hazardous Materials & Abatement Assessment (for Rehab Projects)

- Survey for asbestos, lead paint, mold, PCBs, silica.
- Estimate abatement scope/costs.
- Include permitting and clearances in schedule.

3. Geotechnical & Soils Investigation

- Drill borings; analyze soil composition and stability.
- Evaluate: bearing capacity, liquefaction, subsidence, slope stability, groundwater.
- Provide foundation, grading, pavement, and retaining wall recommendations.

III. INFRASTRUCTURE & UTILITY DUE DILIGENCE

1. Civil Engineering Feasibility

- Preliminary grading and drainage design.
- Stormwater management (SWPPP/NPDES).
- Hydrology & utility capacity studies.

- Identify off-site improvement obligations (ADA, fire access, sidewalks).

2. Utility Coordination & Will-Serve Letters

- Confirm service with providers (electric, gas, water, sewer, telecom).
- Verify nearest connection points and lead times.
- Confirm cost responsibilities for trenching, upgrades, and meters.

3. Traffic & Access Studies

- Traffic Impact Analysis (TIA) if required.
- Verify ingress/egress geometry, emergency vehicle/fire lane compliance.
- Assess parking, ADA access, and public transit availability.

IV. ARCHITECTURAL & PROGRAMMATIC FIT

1. Architectural Test Fits & Conceptual Design

- Engage architect experienced in behavioral health.
- Prepare test fits aligned to program needs.
- Confirm compliance with setbacks, FAR, height, and licensing (DHCS, HCAI).
- Incorporate trauma-informed design principles and clinical workflows.

2. Preliminary Construction Cost Estimates

- ROM estimates including:
    - Site prep and grading.
    - Vertical construction (core/shell, MEP, finishes).
    - Off-site work, hardscape/landscape.
- Factor in:
    - Prevailing wage requirements.
    - Abatement/demolition.

    - Temporary power and stormwater systems.

V. FINANCIAL & OPERATIONAL DUE DILIGENCE

1. Capital Stack & Funding Alignment

- Match costs with grants, tax credits, conventional debt, philanthropy.
- Model reimbursement timing and draw schedules.
- Build full operating pro forma: staffing, insurance, FF&E, reserves.

2. Entitlement & Permitting Timeline Assessment

- Meet with city planning, fire, public works early.
- Map CEQA/NEPA review process.
- Anticipate community hearings and potential NIMBY pushback.
- Build realistic timeline for approvals.

3. Licensing Feasibility

- Align plans with appropriate licensure (RCFE, ARF, CRT, STRTP, SNF, SUD-TX, etc.).
- Verify compliance with plant requirements:
    - Bedroom counts & occupancy ratios.
    - Communal space minimums.
    - Nurse stations, security, and accessibility standards.

CONCLUSION: BUILD ON CERTAINTY, NOT ASSUMPTIONS

The strength of a behavioral health project lies in **certainty, not guesswork.** Comprehensive due diligence:

- Protects against costly unknowns.
- Aligns financing with reality.

- Provides regulators, funders, and operators with confidence.

In a field as **sensitive and regulated** as behavioral health, due diligence is more than a safeguard -it is the **compass guiding capital investment** and the **bridge between vision and execution.**

Build with intention. Build with information. Build with confidence.

> "Chance favors only the prepared mind."
>
> LOUIS PASTEUR

DUE DILIGENCE QUICK REFERENCE CHECKLIST

Behavioral Health Real Estate Development

I. SITE & LEGAL

□ Order **title report** (check easements, liens, CC&Rs, restrictions).
□ Engage **real estate counsel** (zoning, entitlements, contract rights).
□ Obtain **Zoning Verification Letter**; confirm CUP/variances.
□ Commission **ALTA/NSPS survey** (boundaries, easements, encroachments, setbacks).

II. ENVIRONMENTAL & PHYSICAL

□ Conduct **Phase I ESA** (historical land use, hazards).
□ If flagged, perform **Phase II ESA** (soil, groundwater, vapor testing).
□ Complete **hazardous materials survey** (asbestos, lead, mold, PCBs).
□ Schedule **geotechnical investigation** (soil stability, groundwater, slope).

III. INFRASTRUCTURE & UTILITIES

☐ Civil engineering feasibility (grading, drainage, stormwater).
☐ Request **Will-Serve Letters** (electric, gas, water, sewer, telecom).
☐ Confirm **utility capacity & costs** for trenching, upgrades, meters.
☐ Conduct **Traffic Impact Analysis** (ingress/egress, fire access, ADA).

IV. ARCHITECTURAL & PROGRAMMATIC FIT

☐ Develop **test fits** with behavioral health architect.
☐ Align plans with **licensing (DHCS, HCAI)** & trauma-informed design.
☐ Prepare **ROM cost estimates** (site prep, vertical, off-site, soft costs).
☐ Factor **prevailing wage, abatement, and temporary utilities**.

V. FINANCIAL & OPERATIONAL

☐ Build **capital stack** (grants, credits, debt, philanthropy).
☐ Align pro forma with **funding timelines & reimbursement cycles**.
☐ Model **operating budget** (staffing, rent, FF&E, reserves).
☐ Validate **entitlement & permitting timeline** with agencies.
☐ Confirm **licensure feasibility** (RCFE, ARF, CRT, SNF, SUD-TX, etc.).

RULE OF THUMB

Build on certainty, not assumption. Every unchecked box = a future risk.

This detailed breakdown expands on the overview presented earlier. While we previously introduced the six phases of development as a framework, this section provides practical guidance for implementation.

Each phase now includes specific action steps, key players, and potential challenges to navigate. Consider this your tactical playbook for executing the strategic roadmap outlined above.

The following structure offers both depth and clarity:

Phase 1: Concept Planning

- Define the vision and goals of the project.
- Assess community needs and service gaps.
- Develop a preliminary budget and operating plan.
- Engage early advisors: architects, planners, and financial experts.

Outcome: Clear direction and stakeholder alignment.

Key Steps:

- Site Selection & Market Research: Identifying suitable locations based on zoning, accessibility, demand, and economic viability.
- Preliminary Financial Modeling: Estimating development costs, potential revenues, and investment returns.
- Stakeholder Engagement: Consulting with investors, municipal agencies, and community representatives.
- Early Team Formation: Engaging architects, planners, and financial consultants.
- Project Scope Definition: Establishing the intended use, size, and target demographic.

Key Players:

- Owners/Developers: Define project objectives and feasibility.
- Market Analysts: Assess demand and economic conditions.
- Architects & Planners: Provide initial site concepts and massing studies.
- Financial Analysts: Develop preliminary pro formas.

Challenges & Opportunities:

- Challenges: zoning limitations, community pushback, and inaccurate financial assumptions.
- Opportunities: Early engagement with municipal authorities and adaptive reuse of existing sites.

Phase 2: Due Diligence and Feasibility Analysis

- Conduct environmental and geotechnical assessments.
- Verify zoning, land use, and infrastructure capacity.
- Finalize the financial feasibility and risk analysis.

Outcome: Confident site selection and project go/no-go clarity. The due diligence ensures that the proposed site is viable and aids the project team in identifying potential constraints and risks before significant investment is made.

Key Steps:

- Environmental Assessments: Conducting Phase I and II Environmental Site Assessments (ESAs) to identify contamination risks.
- Land Use & Zoning Analysis: Confirming allowable land uses and required approvals.
- Geotechnical and Soil Studies: Evaluating soil stability for structural integrity.
- Utility Assessments: Working with dry utility consultants to determine service availability.
- Will-Serve Letters: Securing commitments from utility providers.
- Preliminary Budgeting & Financing: Refining cost estimates and identifying funding sources.
- Risk Assessment & Exit Strategy: Developing contingency plans for potential obstacles.

Key Players:

- Environmental Consultants: Conduct ESAs and remediation planning.
- Civil Engineers: Assess site infrastructure and drainage.
- Legal Counsel: Ensures compliance with local land use laws.
- Utility Consultants: Confirm service availability.

Challenges & Opportunities:

- Challenges: environmental contamination, restrictive zoning laws, and unanticipated site conditions.
- Opportunities: Incentives for redevelopment and public-private partnerships.

Phase 3: Schematic Design and Entitlements

- Develop early drawings and site plans.
- Submit for entitlements, CUPs, and CEQA review.
- Host community engagement sessions and public hearings.

Outcome: Approved plans that reflect both regulatory needs and community support. This phase involves design development, community outreach, and regulatory compliance.

Key Steps:

- Schematic Design Development: Architects create conceptual site plans, elevations, and layouts.
- Engineering Coordination: Civil, structural, mechanical, and electrical engineers provide input.
- Community Outreach & Public Hearings: Engaging stakeholders and addressing concerns.
- Submitting Entitlement Applications Seeking rezoning, variances, and conditional use permits.

- Regulatory Negotiations & Compliance: Working with city planners and review boards.
- Budget Refinements: Updating financial projections based on entitlement-related costs.

Key Players:

- Architects & Planners: Create schematic designs.
- Attorneys & Lobbyists: Navigate the entitlement process.
- Community Relations Specialists: Manage outreach efforts.

Challenges & Opportunities:

- Challenges: Lengthy approval timelines, community opposition, and unexpected regulatory requirements.
- Opportunities: Collaboration with local authorities to streamline approvals.

Phase 4: Construction Drawings and Permitting

- Finalize blueprints and engineering documents.
- Apply for building, utility, and fire permits.
- Conduct value engineering to maintain scope and budget.
- Outcome: Permit-ready plans with a locked-in construction strategy. Once entitlements are secured, detailed design and permitting commence.

Key Steps:

- Creation of Construction Documents (CDs): Architects and engineers finalize blueprints.
- Permitting Submissions: Coordinating with local agencies for approvals.
- Bid Package Preparation: Developing documentation for contractor selection.

- Pre-Construction Coordination: Reviewing constructability and materials procurement.
- Final Budget Lockdown: Refining financials based on contractor input.

Key Players:

- Architects & Engineers: Produce construction drawings.
- Permit Expediters: Facilitate approvals.
- Project Managers: Coordinate pre-construction activities.

Challenges & Opportunities:

- Challenges: permit delays, design revisions, and rising material costs.
- Opportunities: Value engineering to optimize costs.

Phase 5: General Contractor Selection and Contracting

- Issue RFPs and compare bids.
- Evaluate qualifications, pricing, and schedule.
- Finalize contracts with clear performance terms.

Outcome: A reliable, mission-aligned construction partner. Selecting the right general contractor (GC) is critical to maintaining budget and schedule discipline.

Key Steps:

- Request for Proposal (RFP) Process: Soliciting and evaluating bids.
- Bid Evaluations & Value Engineering: Ensuring cost efficiency.
- Contract Negotiations: Defining terms, schedules, and performance benchmarks.
- Procurement Planning: Identifying long-lead items.

Key Players:

- General Contractors: Oversee construction execution.
- Construction Managers: Manage logistics and scheduling.
- Procurement Specialists: Handle material sourcing.

Challenges & Opportunities:

- Challenges: Finding qualified contractors, rising labor costs.
- Opportunities: Negotiating bulk pricing for materials.

Phase 6: Construction, Commissioning, and Move-In

- Oversee construction execution and quality inspections.
- Complete final walkthroughs and punch lists.
- Obtain certificate of occupancy and prepare for operations.
- Outcome: A licensed, operational facility ready to serve the community. This phase is where the vision becomes reality!

Key Steps:

- MEP Installation: Installing mechanical, electrical, and plumbing systems.
- Inspections and Quality Control: Conducting city inspections and final walkthroughs.
- Final Budget Reconciliation: Closing financials.
- Certificate of Occupancy & Move-In Coordination: Transitioning occupants into the space.

Key Players:

- General Contractors & Subcontractors: Execute construction.
- Inspectors and Compliance Officers: Ensure regulatory adherence.
- Facility Managers: Prepare for occupancy.

Challenges & Opportunities:

Challenges: weather delays, supply chain disruptions, labor shortages.

Opportunities: Implementing sustainability features such as:

- Energy-efficient HVAC systems to reduce operational costs
- Water conservation fixtures and drought-resistant landscaping
- Solar panel installation to offset energy use
- Sustainable building materials for lower environmental impact
- Smart building technologies for optimized resource management
- LEED or WELL certification to demonstrate environmental commitment

CRITICAL LEADERSHIP ROLE IN ALL 6 PHASES: THE ROLE OF THE OWNER'S ADVISOR

Throughout every stage, a skilled Owner's Advisor acts as the central hub, coordinating decisions, managing risks, and maintaining alignment between design intent, budget, and schedule. This role is especially critical in behavioral health, where the stakes are high and the complexity is deep.

BEST PRACTICES FOR SUCCESSFUL STRATEGIC PLANNING

Behavioral health real estate projects succeed when they are grounded in **clarity, collaboration, and discipline**. Strategic planning sets the tone for the entire development lifecycle.

1. START WITH A SHARED VISION

- Define mission, population served, and services offered.
- Establish long-term goals that guide design, site criteria, operations, and finances.
- Translate vision into **design principles, KPIs, and financial benchmarks**.

2. BUILD A STRATEGIC, MULTIDISCIPLINARY TEAM

- Engage SMEs early: real estate developers, clinical planners, architects, engineers, financial analysts, and utility consultants.
- Validate assumptions across **clinical, financial, regulatory, and operational dimensions**.

3. CONDUCT RIGOROUS DUE DILIGENCE

- Complete **title reports, ALTA surveys, zoning analysis, utility access, and geotechnical investigations** before acquisition/design.
- Factor in **licensing pre-checks, FGI/ADA compliance, CEQA/environmental reviews, and AHJ coordination**.
- DBIA data: projects skipping due diligence face a **60% higher risk** of redesign or permit denial.

4. MODEL REALISTIC FINANCIAL SCENARIOS

- Develop **base-case and worst-case pro formas** with escalation factors.
- Define sources/uses of funds and capital stack assumptions.
- Include **5–10% construction contingencies** and operating reserves.
- Build for **financial sustainability**, not just initial feasibility.

5. USE PHASED DECISION-MAKING & RISK REGISTERS

- Phase commitments to de-risk early decisions.
- Maintain a **risk register**, updated weekly with status and responsible parties.
- Treat risk management as **anticipation, not reaction**.

6. ENGAGE STAKEHOLDERS FROM DAY ONE

- Involve **city planning officials, regulators, funders, neighbors, operators, and hospital partners**.
- Early, transparent engagement accelerates approvals and reduces opposition.

7. DOCUMENT EVERYTHING

- Maintain **decision logs, meeting minutes, team charters, and shared digital libraries**.
- Track **schedule, budget, and entitlements** with dashboards.
- Create institutional memory to support handoffs and continuity.

WHY IT MATTERS

Planning failures are costly:

- McKinsey (2022):**70%+ of large-scale construction projects exceed budget** due to incomplete planning and team misalignment.
- In behavioral health, where projects are grant-funded and deadline-driven, **the margin for error is nearly zero**.

By contrast, **integrated planning delivers results**:

- DBIA data:
  - **33% faster delivery**
  - **6–10% lower cost growth**
  - **2.5x higher stakeholder satisfaction**

These aren't theoretical gains -they are the direct result of **front-loaded, collaborative, owner-led strategic planning**.

CONCLUSION: THE POWER OF PREPARATION

Strategic planning is the backbone of successful behavioral health real estate development. In a sector where complexity is high, risk is substantial, and margins for error are narrow, outcomes are determined not by chance, but by preparation, discipline, and alignment. According to the Design-Build Institute of America (DBIA), projects that integrate early planning and collaborative preconstruction practices are completed 33% faster and cost 6% less on average than traditional delivery models. These statistics underscore a fundamental truth: success is designed before it is built.

In behavioral health development, strategic planning isn't an early milestone; it is the foundation upon which the entire project rests. This phase defines scope, aligns teams, and translates a vision into actionable, fundable, and buildable steps. Without comprehensive feasibility modeling, stakeholder engagement, and regulatory review, even the most well-intentioned projects face delays, cost overruns, or licensing failures.

The Owner's Advisor serves as the central force in this orchestration. The Advisor, a true subject matter expert, coordinates diverse disciplines, from architecture and finance to clinical planning and construction, to create harmony between ambition and execution. DBIA's 2023 research confirms that when an Owner's Advisor is engaged during the earliest stages of design, project risk is reduced by 25%, and schedule certainty increases by over 30%.

This level of strategic integration is essential in behavioral health, where facilities must meet demanding codes, serve vulnerable populations, and support long-term operational success.

A missed regulatory requirement or an underestimated cost variable can derail not just a schedule but an entire mission.

FINAL THOUGHTS: FROM PLANNING TO TRANSFORMATION

The chapters ahead will explore how strategic plans evolve into design documents, bid packages, construction milestones, and clinical operations. But, as this chapter affirms, those outcomes are only as strong as their foundation.

Success is cultivated, not assumed. It begins with a disciplined "Owner's Advisor," a team of engaged professionals, a process rooted in real data, and a shared commitment to purpose.

Behavioral health real estate development is not just about bricks and land. It's about creating safe, dignified, and healing environments -environments where human potential can be restored, where care can be delivered with compassion, and where operational sustainability is built into every square foot.

That journey begins not with construction, but with clarity. Not with drawings, but with decisions. And not with hope, but with preparation.

> "The future belongs to those who prepare for it today."
>
> MALCOLM X

Chapter 3

Team Assembly and Leadership **STRUCTURE**

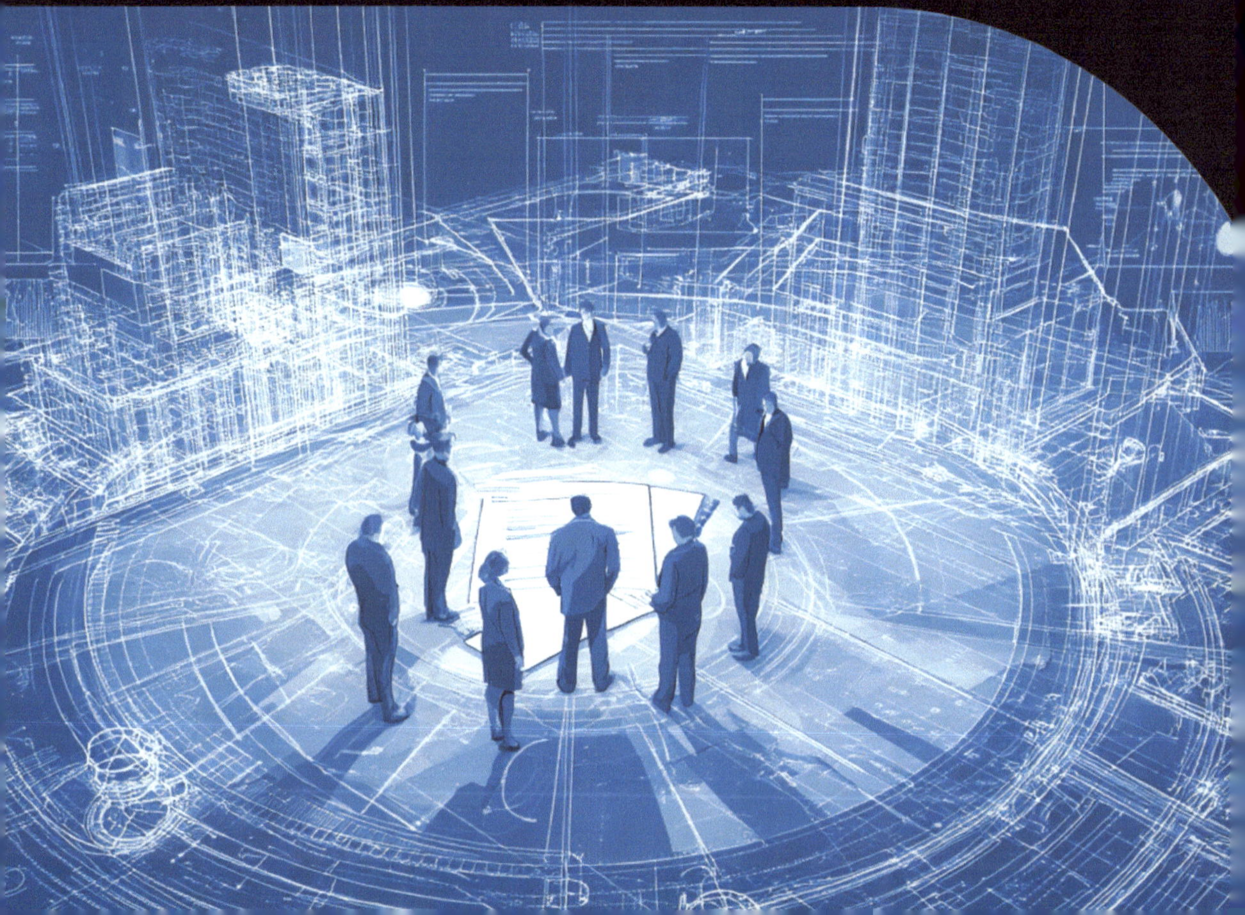

CHAPTER 3
TEAM ASSEMBLY AND LEADERSHIP STRUCTURE

WHAT YOU WILL LEARN IN THIS CHAPTER:

- Defining Core Team Roles: Owner's Advisor, Developer, Architect, Engineer, GC
- Selection Criteria and Procurement Approaches
- Contracting Strategies: Progressive Rapid Delivery, Design-Build, Guaranteed Maximum Price (GMAX)
- The Owner's Representative vs. Owner's Advisor Distinction: Importance of Both!
- Creating Collaborative Team Dynamics and Accountability Models

Breakthroughs in behavioral health infrastructure do not happen in isolation. When capable minds align around a clear aim, the whole becomes greater than the sum of its parts and execution accelerates. For projects with clinical, regulatory, and community dimensions, assemble a circle whose skills complement one another and whose candor sharpens decisions. Set the shared aim, keep a steady cadence, and let the group's intelligence drive momentum through permitting, design, and delivery.

The Owner's Advisor curates this harmony so intent becomes buildable scope, credible schedules, and community trust. Establish a written charter that spells out roles, cadence, and decision rules, then pair it with objective dashboards so the team deals in facts, not assumptions. Bring the right voices in at the right time, and protect the meeting rhythm that keeps issues small and progress visible. The outcome is a team that thinks together and moves together.

In behavioral health real estate development, assembling the right team is the single most important predictor of project success. While strategy and planning establish the vision, it is the human architecture (the roles, relationships, and accountability structures) that turns plans into performance.

Behavioral health projects demand more than routine development expertise. These projects require a team that understands trauma-informed care, healthcare licensure, high-acuity environments, and a public-facing mission. As such, each role must be carefully selected, every relationship purposefully constructed, and the entire structure designed to foster collaboration, trust, and disciplined execution.

In this chapter, we explore the core components of a high-performance project team, from role definition and procurement strategies to the critical leadership distinctions between an Owner's Representative and an Owner's Advisor. We conclude by outlining proven methods to build accountability and collaboration into the DNA of your development team.

FRONT LINE STORY #4. "BUILDING THE DREAM TEAM: A NEW MODEL FOR COLLABORATION"

> "Teamwork is the ability to work together toward a common vision... It is the fuel that allows common people to attain uncommon results."
>
> ANDREW CARNEGIE

I'll never forget the design charrette for a residential facility in Central California. Traditionally, these meetings are a two-way conversation between the architect and the clinical director. This time, I insisted on a third voice at the table: a peer advocate named Marcus, who had experienced homelessness and navigated the very system we were trying to improve. Initially, the dynamic was predictable. The architect laid out a clean, efficient patient intake flow. The therapist countered with needs for privacy and de-escalation zones.

Then Marcus spoke up. He quietly pointed to the floor plan and said, "I see where you're going, but when you first walk in, you're scared. You're made to feel like a number. Here, the first thing you see is a security desk and a long hallway. The message is, 'You are a risk.' What if the first thing you saw was a garden? Or a friendly face offering you water?" The room went silent. In that moment, Marcus's lived experience became more valuable than any blueprint or clinical theory. We threw out the initial layout and started over, designing the entire patient flow around that first moment of contact. We moved the administrative functions to the side and designed a circular, light-filled welcome area centered on a small, therapeutic courtyard. It was a fundamental shift, driven not by a professional, but by the person we were there to serve. That day, we didn't just design a building; we built a team that understood true, human-centered design.

DEFINING CORE TEAM ROLES

A well-balanced and seasoned project team brings together critical expertise across planning, design, construction, compliance, and financing. Each of the core roles listed below brings unique value and carries distinct risks if poorly selected or misaligned.

Defining Core Team Roles: Subject Matter Experts Driving Project Success

A successful behavioral health development project is not built by chance. It is crafted by a disciplined, expert-driven team led by a clear hierarchy of strategic professionals. In this section, we present the most essential players in the development process, ranked in order of influence and importance. Each member of the team brings unique subject matter expertise that, when aligned under a shared vision, propels the project forward with clarity and precision.

1) The Owner: The Mission-Driven Leader

The Owner is the origin of the project's vision and values. They are the financier, decision-maker, and ultimate steward of the project's purpose.

Key Responsibilities:

Define the mission, priorities, and success criteria.

- Approve all major decisions, budgets, and timelines.
- Empower the project team to act on their behalf. An engaged and informed Owner sets the tone for the entire project. Their commitment to quality, community impact, and clinical excellence provides the foundation upon which all other decisions are made.

2) The Real Estate Attorney: The Legal Strategist

The Real Estate Attorney safeguards the project from legal, regulatory, and contractual risk. They ensure that every deal is properly structured, every agreement is enforceable, and every step complies with the complex matrix of real estate and healthcare law.

Key Responsibilities:

- Structure site acquisition, purchase agreements, and land use documents.
- Draft and negotiate contracts with design, construction, and consultant teams.
- Advise on entitlement, leasing, insurance, and regulatory compliance.

This legal expert is a key player from pre-development through closeout, and their counsel helps avoid costly disputes, delays, or vulnerabilities.

3) The Owner's Advisor: The Strategic Integrator

Often the unsung hero, the Owner's Advisor is the Owner's eyes, ears, and strategic guide throughout the project. This subject matter expert offers high-level insight into planning, design, funding, construction, and operations. They serve as the connective tissue between team members, protecting the Owner's interests and ensuring mission alignment at every turn.

Key Responsibilities:

- Guide project delivery strategy (e.g., CMAR, Design-Build, Progressive GMP).
- Advise on team selection, procurement, and scope alignment.
- Facilitate alignment across schedule, scope, budget, and stakeholder priorities.
- Serve as a risk manager and decision-making partner. The Owner's Advisor sees the big picture and the fine print, ensuring long-term sustainability and short-term performance.

4) The Developer: The Financial and Regulatory Navigator

The Developer is the operational engine of the project, coordinating feasibility, finance, entitlement, and predevelopment strategy. In many behavioral health projects, the developer is either a mission-aligned investor or a third-party partner specializing in healthcare facilities.

Key Responsibilities:

- Perform market and financial feasibility analyses.
- Secure public and private funding, tax credits, and grants.
- Lead entitlements, environmental reviews, and community engagement.
- Develop long-term ownership and operating structures.

The Developer brings mastery in real estate finance, local policy, and project logistics. Their work is vital to turning a bold idea into a fundable and approvable project.

5) The Architect: The Vision Translator

The Architect translates operational goals and clinical values into physical form. This expert leads the design process from programming to construction documents, ensuring spaces are functional, beautiful, and healing.

Key Responsibilities:

- Conduct stakeholder workshops and design charrettes.
- Lead architectural programming and conceptual design.
- Coordinate with engineers, consultants, and regulators.
- Ensure adherence to behavioral health design standards. An architect experienced in behavioral health brings specialized knowledge in trauma-informed care environments, ligature resistance, and operational safety. Their expertise influences everything from staff workflows to patient recovery.

6) The Civil Engineer: The Site Solutions Expert

The Civil Engineer transforms a plot of land into a buildable, service-ready site. They are experts in land grading, drainage, utilities, and transportation integration.

Key Responsibilities:

- Conduct site surveys and topographic analysis.
- Design site access, grading, and stormwater systems.
- Coordinate utility infrastructure and "will-serve" letters.
- Support zoning, entitlement, and public works permitting. In behavioral health, civil engineers must account for privacy buffers, therapeutic landscapes, and secure site access. Their early involvement prevents costly surprises during permitting and construction.

7) The General Contractor (GC): The Execution Specialist

The GC brings the building to life. This professional manages labor, materials, subcontractors, inspections, and jobsite safety from groundbreaking to closeout.

Key Responsibilities:

- Prepare and maintain construction schedules.
- Develop budgets, cost estimates, and GMPs.
- Procure subcontractors and materials.
- Ensure construction quality, safety, and compliance.

GCs with behavioral health experience are attuned to specialized facility requirements, patient safety measures, and high-stakes inspections. Their leadership in the field turns ideas into brick-and-mortar healing spaces.

These seven roles form the wellspring leadership structure of every high-performing behavioral health real estate project. When selected with care, aligned with mission, and empowered to collaborate, these subject matter experts ensure that every dollar spent and every decision made serves the goal of lasting impact.

In behavioral health real estate development, assembling the right team is more than a logistical necessity; it is a strategic imperative. Every successful project begins with strong leadership, clear roles, and expert collaboration. At the core of effective project leadership are:

The Owner, who sets the mission and funds the vision.

The Real Estate Attorney, who protects legal integrity and ensures contractual clarity.

The Owner's Advisor, who operationalizes strategy, manages complexity, and aligns the entire team toward successful execution.

The Developer, who runs the day-to-day operations of coordination and execution.

The Owner's Advisor is secondary only to the Owner and Real Estate Attorney in project influence. This role functions as the owner's strategic right hand, deeply embedded in every aspect of the project lifecycle. The Advisor ensures the team is purpose-built, aligned with the mission, and equipped to manage risk across all phases.

Let's explore how each of the core team roles fits into this framework, with the Owner's Advisor serving as the integrator between them.

A successful behavioral health project is driven by the strength, synergy, and structure of its core team. These professionals are not just executing tasks; they are shaping environments that will support healing, dignity, and long-term community well-being. Each role carries unique responsibilities and contributes to a cohesive project ecosystem.

CORE TEAM ROLES IN BEHAVIORAL HEALTH REAL ESTATE DEVELOPMENT

Behavioral health facility projects demand the **integration of vision, strategy, and technical expertise**. The following core roles represent the brain, backbone, and muscle of a successful project team.

DEVELOPER

The developer serves as the **central leader and visionary**, ultimately accountable for project success.

Key Responsibilities

- Identify and secure the project site
- Conduct or oversee feasibility studies
- Secure capital and manage investor relationships
- Lead entitlement and permitting strategies
- Align design, construction, and operations with mission-driven goals

Behavioral Health-Specific Competencies

- Understanding of **Medi-Cal reimbursement models**
- Knowledge of **state and county behavioral health funding streams** (e.g., MHSA in California)
- Awareness of **clinical programming and licensure requirements**

Developers must balance **bold vision with practical execution**, creating partnerships and systems that sustain outcomes.

ARCHITECT

The architect translates **clinical intent and operational goals** into healing environments.

Key Responsibilities

- Facilitate early design charrettes and stakeholder visioning
- Produce conceptual, schematic, and construction documents
- Integrate **trauma-informed design** and **biophilic principles**
- Coordinate engineering consultants
- Ensure compliance with **ADA, life safety, fire code, and licensing** requirements

Behavioral Health-Specific Competencies

- Prior experience in **inpatient and outpatient behavioral health** design
- Understanding of **ligature resistance, safety zoning, and patient dignity**
- Capacity to lead **inclusive, collaborative design processes**

ENGINEERS (CIVIL, STRUCTURAL, MEP, LOW-VOLTAGE)

Engineers ensure the **technical feasibility, safety, and compliance** of facility systems.

Disciplines and Focus

- **Civil**: Site grading, stormwater, roads, utilities
- **Structural**: Load-bearing systems, seismic design, lateral stability
- **MEP**: HVAC, electrical, plumbing, fire protection
- **Low-Voltage**: Nurse call, security, IT cabling, audiovisual systems

Behavioral Health-Specific Sensitivities

- Infection control via **negative-pressure HVAC zones**
- **Acoustic dampening** for privacy
- **Redundant power systems** for life-safety needs

GENERAL CONTRACTOR (GC)

The GC makes the project real -overseeing **labor, procurement, safety, and schedule**.

Key Responsibilities

- Preconstruction pricing and scheduling
- Subcontractor selection and bid leveling
- Jobsite safety and regulatory compliance
- Quality control and constructability feedback
- Coordination of inspections, commissioning, and closeout

Behavioral Health-Specific Competencies

- Familiarity with **anti-ligature hardware and finishes**

- Sensitivity to **confidentiality, security, and patient flow**
- Knowledge of **OSHPD/DSA/AHJ-specific inspection protocols**

OWNER'S ADVISOR

The Owner's Advisor is the **strategic leader and trusted partner** guiding the project at the highest level.

Key Responsibilities

- Assemble the project team and guide procurement
- Advise on **delivery models** (CMAR, GMAX, Design-Build)
- Lead **budget, risk, and schedule strategy sessions**
- Ensure alignment with **clinical, financial, and operational goals**
- Monitor performance and resolve high-level conflicts

This role is especially critical in behavioral health, where decisions affect **vulnerable populations and regulated systems**.

CONSTRUCTION MANAGER FOR OWNER (CM FOR OWNER)

The CM for Owner provides **technical oversight of the GC** -a translator and watchdog during construction.

Key Responsibilities

- Review contractor schedules and sequencing
- Evaluate RFIs, submittals, and change orders
- Verify cost estimates and GMAX compliance
- Monitor construction quality and safety
- Liaise between GC and Owner on construction issues

In behavioral health, where operational disruptions are costly and dangerous, this role is **invaluable for safeguarding design intent and budget**.

SELECTION CRITERIA AND PROCUREMENT APPROACHES

Selecting the right professionals is **as critical as site selection**.

Core Selection Criteria

- Experience with behavioral health or healthcare projects
- Familiarity with **local entitlement/permitting authorities**
- Knowledge of **codes and safety standards**
- Track record of **cost transparency and risk management**
- Team chemistry and collaborative practices

Procurement Models

- **RFQ (Request for Qualifications):** Shortlists firms based on experience.
- **RFP (Request for Proposals):** Includes fee proposals, project approach, and team bios.
- **Interviews & Scoring Matrix:** Structured evaluation with weighted criteria.

Contracting Strategies

- **Progressive Rapid Delivery**: Overlapping design/construction phases; early GC engagement.
- **Design-Build (DB)**: Single-entity responsibility; fewer disputes; faster delivery.
- **Guaranteed Maximum Price (GMAX)**: Cost cap with transparency; incentivizes collaboration.

The **Owner's Advisor** helps determine which model best fits the project's risk, complexity, and funding structure.

OWNER'S REPRESENTATIVE VS. OWNER'S ADVISOR

Owner's Representative

- Day-to-day project administrator
- Manages RFI/submittal logs
- Coordinates meeting minutes and task tracking
- Acts as liaison with design/construction teams

Owner's Advisor

- Strategic partner with executive insight
- Guides procurement, risk, and contracting strategy
- Advises on team selection and performance
- Aligns all decisions with **mission and long-term success**

Both roles are complementary:

- The **Advisor sets strategy**.
- The **Representative manages execution**.

CREATING COLLABORATIVE TEAM DYNAMICS

A strong team is more than skilled individuals -it is a **cohesive, mission-driven system**.

Foundations of Collaboration

- **Shared Mission:** Teams must understand the "why."
- **Integrated Kick-Offs:** All disciplines aligned early.
- **Clear Communication Protocols:** Defined cadence, escalation, and documentation.

Accountability Structures

- **RACI Matrix:** Defines responsibility and authority.
- **Phase Gates:** Formal checkpoints for approval.
- **Performance Dashboards:** Real-time tracking of budget, schedule, risks.

Conflict Management

- Pre-established resolution protocols
- Neutral facilitation for critical issues
- Document all decisions and assumptions

Culture Building

- Celebrate milestones (big and small)
- Recognize individual contributions
- Foster **psychological safety** in team meetings

CONCLUSION

By clearly defining **roles**, selecting partners with **intention**, and cultivating **collaborative culture**, behavioral health real estate teams build more than facilities -they build **safe, dignified environments of care**.

> "The function of leadership is to produce more leaders, not more followers."
>
> RALPH NADER

FRONT LINE STORY #5: LEADERSHIP LESSONS: "MISSION OVER EGO"

On one of our most ambitious projects, we hit a wall. The lead architect, a renowned designer, had proposed a stunning two-story glass atrium as the facility's central feature. The clinical director, however, was vehemently opposed, arguing that the design created impossible sightline challenges and acoustic issues that would be detrimental to trauma-informed care. The debate became personal, egos became entrenched, and the project ground to a halt for two weeks. The team was divided, and morale was plummeting.

My role as the Owner's Advisor was not to be a judge but a facilitator. I called a meeting with just the two of them, away from the pressures of the larger group. Instead of rehashing the debate, I put the project's one-page mission statement on the table between us. It was a simple document outlining our commitment to creating a "sanctuary for healing, safety, and recovery." I asked a simple question: "Looking at this, how do we honor both visionary design and clinical safety?" I didn't ask who was right; I asked what served the mission.

The shift was immediate. The conversation moved from "my design" and "my concerns" to "our mission." They started sketching on a whiteboard together, and within an hour, they had co-designed a new concept: a series of smaller, interconnected single-story pavilions with clerestory windows that brought in natural light without sacrificing privacy or safety. It was an elegant, effective solution. The experience was a crucial reminder that strong leadership isn't about having the best idea; it's about creating a space where the best idea can emerge by consistently bringing the team back to its shared purpose.

CLOSING THOUGHTS

Team assembly is not simply an administrative task; it is the act of building your project's nervous system. Every decision the team makes, from procurement model to conflict resolution plan, shapes how your project will function under pressure.

In the next chapter, we turn our attention to the Owner's Advisor in greater detail, unpacking how this key role can guide strategy, coordination, and execution across every phase of development.

Chapter 4

The **OWNER'S ADVISOR**: Strategic Leadership at the Core

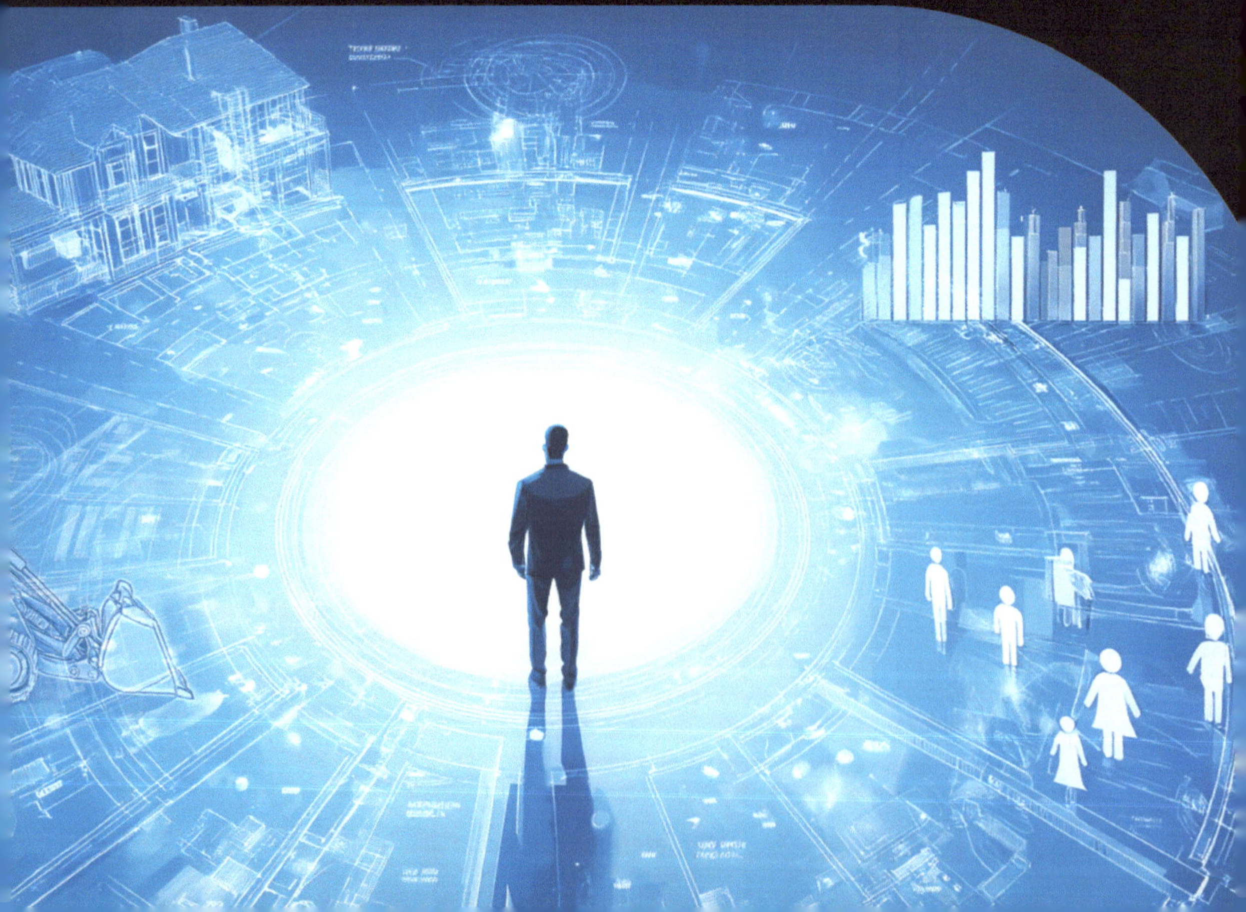

CHAPTER 4
THE OWNER'S ADVISOR, STRATEGIC LEADERSHIP

WHAT YOU WILL LEARN IN THIS CHAPTER:

- The Secret Key: Owner's Advisor as the Ultimate Integrator
- Tactical Influence in Pre-Development and Team Coordination
- Advocacy for Client Mission, Schedule, Scope, and Budget
- Leadership in Decision Making and Performance Management
- Case Studies of Success Led by Owner's Advisors

CHAPTER OVERVIEW

Successful behavioral health real estate development demands more than funding and blueprints. It requires a synchronized effort of experts, guided by a unifying vision and executed with clarity, discipline, and strategy. At the center of this orchestration stands the Owner's Advisor.a seasoned subject matter expert and the project's strategic integrator.

This chapter explores the indispensable role of the Owner's Advisor, their professional background, strategic functions, and the measurable outcomes they produce. Whether navigating community resistance, ensuring regulatory compliance, or safeguarding the Owner's vision, the Owner's Advisor is the essential driver behind mission-aligned, on-time, and on-budget delivery.

Leadership and accurate thinking make the Owner's Advisor the project's nerve center. Make clear decisions under uncertainty. Anchor them in facts that hold up in public and clinical forums. In behavioral health development, this role protects mission, schedule, scope, and budget by creating shared clarity when pressure rises.

Build governance people can follow. Stand up decision logs, stoplight dashboards, and a weekly forum where open items become closed items. Use RACI for the hard calls. Align risk, entitlements, and funding calendars so choices land on time with evidence.

FRONT LINE STORY #6. THE INTEGRATOR ROLE: BRIDGING SILOS

> "The key to successful leadership today is influence, not authority."
>
> KEN BLANCHARD

Throughout my career, I have embraced the role of a strategic servant leader, understanding that every project requires a delicate balance of coordination and collaboration. A significant realization has been the importance of acting as an integrator between teams. In various projects, I have often stepped in to bridge communication gaps, particularly when clinical and construction teams struggled to align their goals. By serving as a translator and facilitator, I have ensured that programmatic objectives align seamlessly with spatial requirements, thus avoiding costly redesigns and delays. This integrative approach has not only saved resources but also fostered a culture of collaboration and mutual respect.

A pivotal moment occurred during a budget negotiation where I advocated to preserve a therapeutic outdoor space that was at risk of being cut from the project. By building a strong case grounded in clinical return on investment (ROI), my team and I successfully championed its inclusion. Today, that courtyard is celebrated as the heart of the facility, a space where staff and patients alike find solace and connection. This experience reinforced my belief that advocacy in action is a fundamental aspect of strategic leadership.

My journey has included financial successes and failures, scheduling conflicts, and permitting challenges. Throughout, I have learned that most obstacles are fundamentally human in nature. The key to overcoming these challenges lies in effective communication and a deep understanding of the diverse players and processes involved. When we work together harmoniously, we can deliver the real estate facilities society desperately needs.

> "The Owner's Advisor is not a luxury; it's the key to success in complex behavioral health developments."
>
> DBIA

THE SECRET KEY: OWNER'S ADVISOR AS THE ULTIMATE INTEGRATOR

The Owner's Advisor is the bridge between vision and execution. While the Owner sets the mission and the Real Estate Attorney ensures legal protection, the Advisor unites the full project ecosystem, ensuring alignment across clinical, financial, architectural, operational, and regulatory domains.

Key Integrative Functions:

- Guides planning, procurement, and preconstruction strategy
- Maintains alignment across schedule, scope, and budget
- Acts as a translator between technical teams and owner intent
- Drives execution through structured decision-making and performance management
- Balances technical feasibility with long-term operational functionality

Real-World Example: In one behavioral health campus project, the Owner's Advisor synchronized over 14 subconsultants, coordinated three government funding streams, and ensured entitlements were secured in parallel with design progression, saving five months of development time and providing 10X savings and value.

Unlike project managers focused on tasks, the Owner's Advisor is responsible for strategic orchestration, stakeholder integration, and holistic quality control. Their oversight ensures the Owner's intent is not only preserved but enhanced by the decisions made throughout the project.

The Benefits of an Experienced Owner's Advisor

- Stronger project outcomes and long-term impact
- Increased cost control and value optimization
- Greater team cohesion and reduced conflict
- Improved public engagement and stakeholder trust
- Strategic continuity through leadership transitions
- Faster issue resolution and decision velocity
- Better regulatory readiness and licensing outcomes

THE ROLE OF THE OWNER'S ADVISOR: A MULTIFACETED STRATEGIC LEADER

The Owner's Advisor serves as the **integrator of vision, operations, compliance, and execution** -a role that goes beyond oversight to shape mission-driven success in behavioral health development.

CORE FUNCTIONS OF THE OWNER'S ADVISOR

Vision Alignment & Strategic Leadership

- Translate mission into **measurable goals and operational KPIs**
- Ensure design and delivery approach supports **clinical objectives**

- Advise on **adaptability, sustainability, and post-occupancy performance**

Stakeholder Coordination & Engagement

- Lead collaboration across **design, construction, finance, and operations**
- Facilitate **planning sessions, town halls, and design charrettes**
- Maintain alignment with **decision logs, stakeholder matrices, and phased feedback**

Budget Oversight & Financial Stewardship

- Develop and maintain **detailed cost models** across all phases
- Facilitate **funding compliance** and grant reporting
- Analyze cost impacts of design decisions and change orders

Quality Assurance & Compliance

- Align designs with **AHJ, ADA, FGI, OSHPD, and state licensing requirements**
- Coordinate **agency pre-application meetings, code reviews, and walkthroughs**
- Oversee **third-party peer reviews, mock-ups, and equipment integration**

Risk Management & Tactical Problem-Solving

- Maintain a **living risk register** with owner-approved strategies
- Lead **design resolution and constructability reviews**
- Anticipate conflicts such as **staff workflows, security, or acoustics**

Post-Completion & Operational Transition

- Establish **training schedules, operational checklists, and FF&E integration**
- Lead **move-in coordination** and emergency preparedness scenarios
- Facilitate **post-occupancy evaluations, warranty tracking, and improvement cycles**

CHALLENGES NAVIGATED BY THE OWNER'S ADVISOR

- **Complex Regulatory Landscape:** Aligns planning with licensing, permitting, and environmental timelines
- **Behavioral Health Design Needs:** Ensures ligature resistance, trauma-informed care, and visual privacy
- **Stakeholder Diversity:** Balances multi-agency funding and cross-functional priorities
- **Public Relations:** Builds trust through grassroots engagement and communication campaigns

STRATEGIES FOR SUCCESS

- **Early Engagement:** Join at pre-feasibility to align **scope, policy, and funding**
- **Integrated Team Building:** Procure teams with **cultural fit, proven expertise, and values alignment**
- **Technology Enablement:** Use **dashboards, BIM tools, and real-time budget tracking**
- **Evidence-Based Design:** Link design to measurable outcomes (e.g., fewer incidents, higher staff retention)
- **Transparent Communication:** Establish **escalation protocols, RACI matrices, and decision logs**

PROFESSIONAL PROFILE: THE MODERN OWNER'S ADVISOR

Credentials

- MBA, MRED, or MS in Healthcare Administration
- PMP, CCM, or LEED AP certifications
- Licensed contractor or registered architect (preferred in design-build contexts)
- Background in both **healthcare operations and real estate development**

Core Competencies

- Strategic Planning & Programming
- Financial Forecasting & Capital Planning
- Health Code & Licensing Navigation
- Regulatory Affairs & Stakeholder Mediation
- Organizational Leadership & Communication

Case Studies in Action

Case Study 1: Urban Behavioral Health Hospital

- Challenge: Tight site, zoning resistance, and budget constraints.
- Advisor Impact: Led early feasibility analysis, design workshops with city agencies, and phased entitlements.
- Result: Completed two months early, under budget, with strong neighborhood support and high operational readiness.

Case Study 2: Crisis Stabilization Unit (CSU)

- Challenge: 10-month delivery timeline tied to grant expiration.

- Advisor Impact: Accelerated design permitting, secured early contractor engagement, and resolved fire authority objections.
- Result: Achieved state licensing with no corrections, protecting $8M in behavioral health funding.

Case Study 3: Integrated Behavioral Health Campus

- Challenge: Multiple funding sources, staffing shortages, and executive turnover.
- Advisor Impact: Maintained continuity, navigated seven agency audits, and fast-tracked clinical staff onboarding.
- Result: Fully operational 90 days post-Certificate of Occupancy (C of O); 92% staff retention after one year.

LIFECYCLE MANAGEMENT: FROM VISION TO ACTIVATION

Pre-Development

- Visioning, programming, and feasibility modeling
- Site selection and entitlement pre-check
- Stakeholder engagement framework development

Design Phase

- Clinical adjacencies and space planning validation
- Consultant scope negotiation and coordination protocols
- Pre-permit review and cost estimating alignment

Construction Phase

- Weekly Owner, Architect, Contractor (OAC) meetings, submittal and RFI tracking
- GMP validation, change order mitigation, and field observations

- Licensure preparation and inspection coordination

Post-Completion

- Punch list closeout and commissioning review
- Move-in support, staff training, and documentation turnover
- Post-occupancy review and facilities performance analysis

CONCLUSION: THE OWNER'S ADVISOR AS THE STRATEGIC CATALYST

The Owner's Advisor is not a support role; it is a strategic leadership role. From initial site assessment to post-occupancy evaluation, they are the connective tissue that binds together the many moving parts of behavioral health facility development. With mastery in design thinking, operational planning, and regulatory navigation, the Owner's Advisor ensures every decision serves the greater mission.

Data from the Design-Build Institute of America (DBIA) supports this vital role. According to DBIA industry studies:

- Projects that include an early-engaged Owner's Advisor experience up to 30% faster delivery.
- Owner satisfaction scores increase by 40% when the Owner's Advisor is actively involved in cross-disciplinary coordination.
- The average cost overrun risk decreases by up to 20% in behavioral health projects when the Owner's Advisor leads early feasibility and scope alignment.

In an industry plagued by uncertainty, complexity, and constant regulatory change, the Owner's Advisor brings strategy, foresight, and discipline to every phase:

- They convert complexity into clarity.
- They turn fragmented decisions into coordinated execution.
- They transform vision into healing, operational, and architectural success.

With pressure mounting across healthcare systems and behavioral health infrastructure in high demand, the Owner's Advisor ensures projects stay focused, agile, and mission-aligned. Their involvement mitigates risk, enhances design quality, accelerates approvals, and fosters trust across all stakeholders.

Engaging the right Owner's Advisor means more than just adding a team member; it means securing a strategic partner. A leader who can span silos, translate intent into execution, and anticipate challenges before they become problems. The Owner's Advisor becomes the single most valuable asset in turning behavioral health development into high-impact, community-serving success.

> "A great Owner's Advisor doesn't just manage projects. They cultivate success from the ground up and long after doors open."
>
> RICHARD VASQUEZ, OWNER

In the chapters that follow, we will explore how the Owner's Advisor supports procurement, construction administration, and facility activation, guiding every step from strategy to operation with precision, purpose, and a commitment to quality outcomes.

Chapter 5

FINANCING Behavioral Health Infrastructure

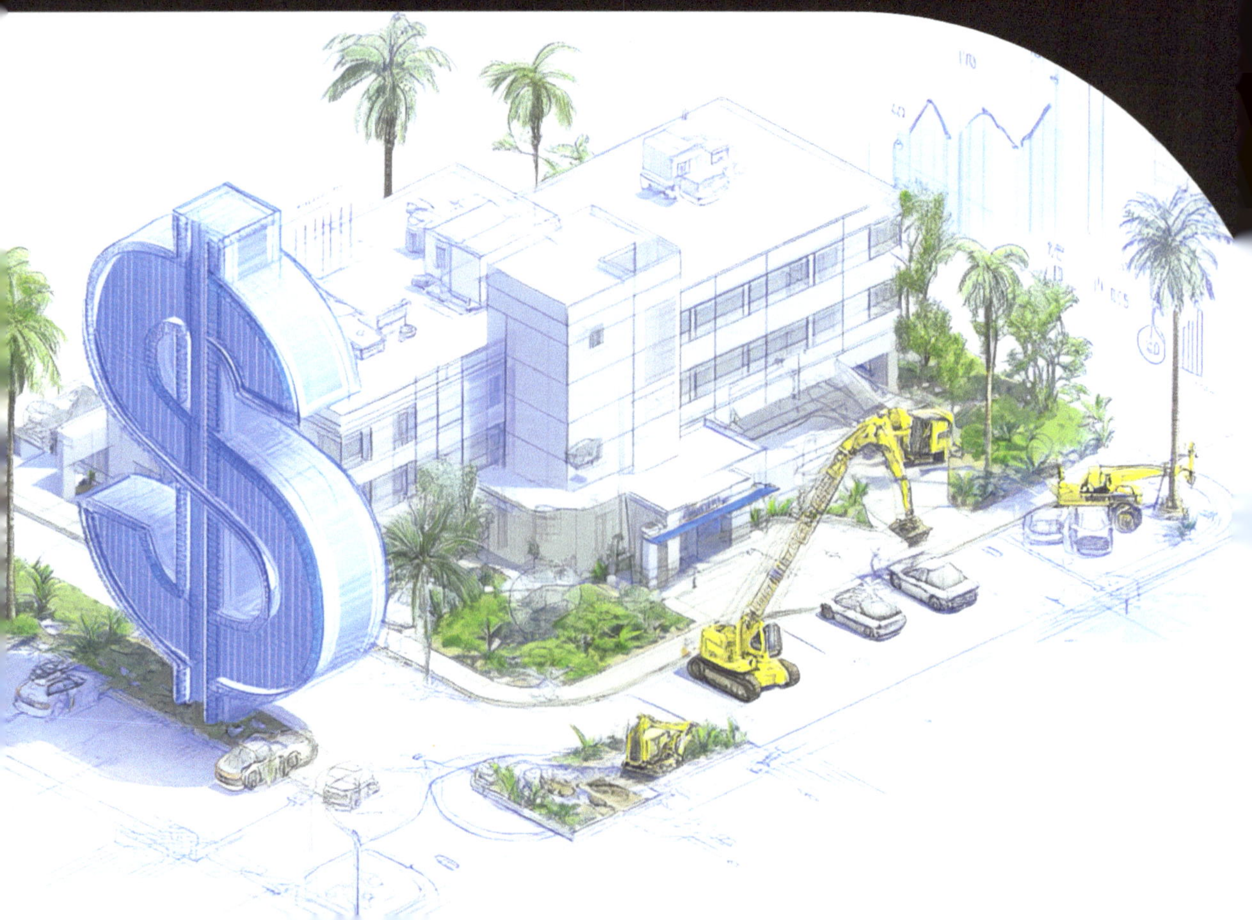

CHAPTER 5
FINANCING BEHAVIORAL HEALTH INFRASTRUCTURE

WHAT YOU WILL LEARN IN THIS CHAPTER

- Capital Planning and Early Feasibility
- Funding Sources and Capital Stacks
- Cost Estimating and Financial Contingency Planning
- Owner's Reserves and Cash Flow Management
- Grant Compliance, Philanthropy, and Debt Structuring
- Fiduciary Best Practices and Risk Management

CHAPTER OVERVIEW

Financing behavioral health facilities is one of the most complex and critical aspects of real estate development. Without the right capital plan, even the best-designed facility may never break ground. This chapter explores the full lifecycle of financial planning and execution, from early feasibility modeling and cost estimating, to assembling a capital stack, to managing contingencies and ensuring fiscal stewardship throughout the life of the project.

Behavioral health projects face unique financing challenges: longer permitting cycles, specialized construction requirements, and complex licensing mandates.

But the upside is equally significant: life-changing care delivered to communities that need it most.

Applied faith and decision drive financing forward when variables are messy. Set a direction, choose a path, and move. Pair confidence with discipline. In behavioral health projects that blend grants, debt, and philanthropy, teams win by deciding decisively and iterating with data.

Turn mindset into a living capital plan. Build the capital stack with scenarios, map cash flows to milestones, and maintain a risk log that drives outreach and backup options. Sync to grant and bond calendars. Tie draws to progress so the schedule keeps cash healthy.

> "Real estate cannot be lost or stolen, nor can it be carried away. Purchased with common sense, paid for in full, and managed with reasonable care, it is about the safest investment in the world."
>
> FRANKLIN D. ROOSEVELT

FRONT LINE STORY #7. CREATIVE FINANCING SOLUTIONS

We had a project on the line: a 30-bed supportive housing facility for individuals with co-occurring disorders. The state grant was secured and we had a motivated developer, but we were facing a $2 million gap in our capital stack. Conventional lenders were hesitant due to the specialized nature of the facility. The project was at risk of collapse.

Instead of giving up, we got creative. Our financial consultant, an expert in mission-driven projects, proposed a layered strategy. First, we applied for New Markets Tax Credits (NMTC), a federal program designed to spur investment in low-income communities. Securing the allocation was a competitive, painstaking process, but it covered nearly half of our gap. Next, we approached a local philanthropic foundation that had never funded capital projects before. We didn't ask for a grant; instead, we framed it as a high-impact social investment, showing them how the facility would reduce emergency room visits and create long-term community stability. They came in with a major contribution. The final piece was a small bridge loan from a Community Development Financial Institution (CDFI), which provided the last bit of capital needed to start construction. By weaving together three unconventional funding sources, we didn't just fill a gap; we built a coalition of partners who were invested in our mission. It was a masterclass in how creative financing is really about creative partnership-building.

BEST PRACTICES IN FINANCING BEHAVIORAL HEALTH DEVELOPMENT

Applied faith and decision drive financing forward when variables are messy. Set a direction, choose a path, and move. Pair confidence with discipline. In behavioral health projects that blend grants, debt, and philanthropy, teams win by deciding decisively and iterating with data.

Turn mindset into a living capital plan. Build the capital stack with scenarios, map cash flows to milestones, and maintain a risk log that drives outreach and backup options. Sync to grant and bond calendars. Tie draws to progress so the schedule keeps cash healthy.

1. Capital Planning and Early Feasibility

Before a site is acquired or a design is drawn, project sponsors must conduct a comprehensive financial feasibility analysis.

Best Practices Include:

- Develop a pro forma that includes construction, FF&E, soft costs, and escalation.
- Align budget assumptions with programming scope and staffing model.
- Validate target rents, service contracts, or reimbursement pathways for financial sustainability.

Key Insight: Projects that complete a third-party financial feasibility study during predevelopment are 2.4 times more likely to close on capital commitments within 12 months (Urban Institute, 2022).

2. Funding Sources and Capital Stacks

Behavioral health facilities are typically financed through blended capital structures. These may include:

- State grants (e.g., California's Behavioral Health Continuum Infrastructure Program (BHCIP))
- Tax-exempt bonds or municipal financing
- Low-Income Housing Tax Credits (LIHTC) for co-located supportive housing
- Philanthropic contributions
- Bank debt or NMTC/HTC allocations

Capital Stack Design Considerations:

- Prioritize non-dilutive funding (grants, etc.) early in the project timeline.
- Structure tranches to align with the construction draw schedule.
- Plan for debt service coverage ratio (DSCR) requirements in operations.

Statistic: Projects with a layered funding structure are 37% more likely to reach financial close if led by a dedicated financial consultant or capital advisor (National Council for Behavioral Health, 2021).

3. Cost Estimating and Financial Contingency Planning

Accurate and realistic cost estimating is foundational to financial stability. Underestimating costs can create mid-project crises; overestimating can delay approvals or funding awards.

Best Practices Include:

- Conduct milestone cost estimates at 30%, 60%, and 90% design stages.
- Incorporate market data for material/labor escalation.

- Include allowances for FF&E, AV, security systems, and IT infrastructure.

Contingency Planning:

- Hard Cost Contingency: 5-10% of total construction costs, depending on project complexity.
- Soft Cost Contingency: 3-5% for professional fees, permitting delays, and entitlements.
- Escalation Reserve: 5-7% to account for volatile labor and material costs.

Result: According to DBIA (2023), behavioral health projects with formal contingency frameworks have 41% fewer change orders and 32% lower cost overruns.

4. Owner's Reserve and Cash Flow Management

The Owner must maintain adequate liquidity to manage unexpected expenses and protect project viability.

Owner Reserve Guidelines:

- Carry an unrestricted reserve equal to at least 3-6 months of operating expenses.
- Establish a Construction Risk Reserve to cover delays in funding draws.
- Maintain cash equivalents to absorb non-reimbursable costs or scope changes.

Cash Flow Monitoring Tools:

- Implement monthly draw projections based on actuals and upcoming trades.
- Use financial dashboards to track burn rate, invoice processing, and lender reporting.

Impact: Projects with a dedicated cash flow manager and reserve fund achieve 23%

faster loan draws and reduce vendor payment disputes by 28% (Construction Finance Management Association, 2022).

5. Grant Compliance, Philanthropy, and Debt Structuring

Grants and donations are often the lifeblood of nonprofit-led projects. They require strict compliance and tracking.

Best Practices:

- Match grant disbursement schedules to construction cash flow needs.
- Track restricted vs. unrestricted funds using project accounting software.
- Engage a CPA or compliance consultant to manage state and federal reporting.

Philanthropy Tips:

- Create naming opportunities tied to capital milestones.
- Use donor walls, storytelling, and program sponsorships to encourage engagement.
- Leverage foundation challenge grants to unlock matching donations.

Debt Strategy:

- Negotiate terms with an emphasis on interest-only periods during construction.
- Evaluate the impact of DSCR on facility operations and long-term financial health.

6. Fiduciary Best Practices and Risk Management

Financial stewardship is a fiduciary responsibility. Behavioral health infrastructure projects often involve public funds, and transparency is essential.

Best Practices Include:

- Maintain clear audit trails for all expenditures.
- Use third-party fund control or construction lenders for draw validation.
- Conduct quarterly budget vs. actual variance analysis.
- Document all budget decisions and funding reallocations.

Outcome: Projects with a formalized financial governance structure are 39% more likely to complete on budget and within the original draw schedule (Brookings Institution, 2021).

FRONT LINE STORY8. FINANCIAL CHALLENGES OVERCOME

> "A nickel ain't worth a dime anymore."
>
> YOGI BERRA

Every developer dreads the call from the geotechnical engineer. For us, it came three weeks into excavation for a new detox center. They had discovered a large pocket of contaminated soil, a remnant from a gas station that had occupied the site decades ago. The remediation cost was staggering: an unbudgeted $800,000 expense that threatened to derail the entire project. Panic set in among the stakeholders.

This is where disciplined financial planning pays off. Our first line of defense was the 10% hard-cost contingency we had built into the pro forma. It was designed for exactly this kind of unforeseen event. It covered more than half the cost, but we still had a significant shortfall. Next, we immediately initiated a value engineering review. Working with the architect and contractor, we identified non-essential design elements (high-end finishes and elaborate landscaping that could be simplified without compromising the clinical function or safety of the facility. Finally, we had a transparent, honest conversation with our general contractor. Because we had built a strong, trust-based relationship, we were able to negotiate a shared-risk approach where they absorbed a small portion of the cost in exchange for timeline flexibility. By combining our contingency fund, strategic cost-cutting, and a strong partnership, we navigated a potential catastrophe and kept the project on track. It was a powerful lesson that financial resilience isn't just about having reserves; it's about having a plan and the relationships to execute it.

> "Great care requires great infrastructure. Great infrastructure requires smart, sustainable financing."
>
> CA. GOVERNOR GAVIN NEWSOM

FINAL THOUGHT: BUILD THE NUMBERS BEHIND THE MISSION

Great behavioral health facilities don't begin with blueprints; they begin with financial vision and planning. The work of healing requires the infrastructure of trust, and that starts with knowing how every dollar supports every square foot.

The most resilient projects are those that forecast clearly, plan conservatively, and execute with transparency. A thoughtful capital strategy isn't just about delivering a building; it's about protecting its future, honoring its mission, and ensuring it will serve generations to come.

> "Finance is not just math; it's the mission in numbers."
>
> BRIAN JONES

PART TWO
FROM CONCEPT THRU PERMITTING

Chapter 6

SITE SELECTION and Location Strategy

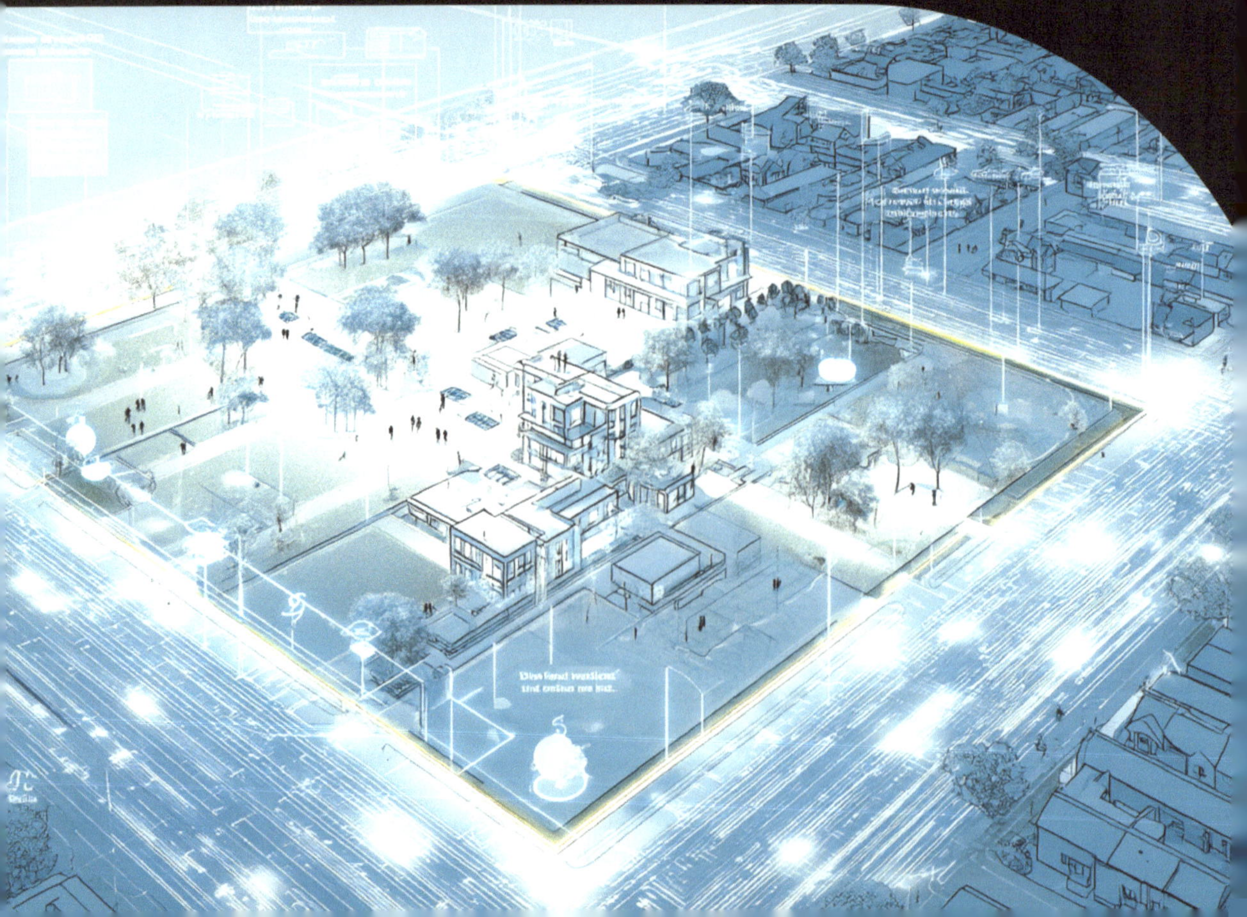

CHAPTER 6
SITE SELECTION: LAYING THE GROUNDWORK FOR SUCCESS

This chapter explores best practices in site selection with a focus on due diligence, feasibility analysis, zoning navigation, and sustainable planning. New development and adaptive reuse both require rigorous investigation into the buildability of land and structures. Central to this process is the Owner's Advisor, a subject matter expert who brings strategic clarity, technical oversight, and coordination excellence to the critical decision-making moments that determine project success.

WHAT YOU WILL LEARN IN THIS CHAPTER:

- Site Analysis Factors
- Feasibility, Chances for Success, & Sustainability
- Site and Structure Due Diligence for Buildability
- Addressing the Challenges of Zoning and Land Use
- Overview of Zoning Laws and Land Use Regulations in California
- Strategies for Overcoming Bureaucratic Hurdles in Real Estate Development
- Case Studies of Successful Navigation of Zoning Challenge

CHAPTER OVERVIEW

The success of a behavioral health rehabilitation facility is deeply rooted in the strategic selection of its site. This single decision has cascading effects on access, entitlements, regulatory approvals, long-term operational efficiency, cost control, and community impact. A well-selected site promotes patient access, stakeholder alignment, and environmental sustainability. A poorly vetted site can derail timelines, inflate budgets, and jeopardize licensing.

Accurate thinking and specialized knowledge make site selection a clinical and operational decision, not just a deal. Separate facts from opinions and test assumptions in the field. For behavioral health, success favors quiet, safe, accessible locations with clear paths through zoning and neighbors who can say yes.

Operationalize with a site scoring matrix that weights clinical fit, zoning, utilities, safety, and community context. Run diligence early. Drive routes at shift-start and shift-end times. Bring planning and licensing into the review so the eventual operator can succeed.

FRONT LINE STORY#9. SITE SELECTION STORY: BEYOND THE BOTTOM LINE

We were scouting a site for a new residential treatment facility, and on paper, the property was perfect. It was centrally located, zoned correctly, and priced to move. The seller was motivated, and our initial pro forma looked promising. But a site isn't just a set of data points on a spreadsheet. It's a future environment for healing.

I decided to visit the location at different times of the day. During the 9 a.m. lull, it was quiet. But when I returned at 5 p.m., the problem became clear. The property was adjacent to a major freeway, and the rush-hour traffic created a constant, percussive roar that vibrated through the ground. I stood there, picturing a resident in therapy, a veteran grappling with PTSD, or a teen in crisis, and imagined their recovery being punctuated by the shriek of tires and the rumble of engines. It was an environment of agitation, not calm. The data said "yes," but the reality of the place said "no."

We walked away from the deal, much to the broker's confusion. A week later, while driving through a quieter, overlooked part of the county, I spotted a series of vacant, single-story medical offices, relics from the 1980s. The property was underutilized and set back from the main road, surrounded by mature trees. It wasn't on any broker's hot sheet, but it was peaceful. We tracked down the owner, and what began as a long shot turned into our next project: a facility designed with tranquility at its core. That experience solidified a core principle for me: for behavioral health, the most valuable asset of a property isn't its price, but its potential to foster peace.

THE ART AND SCIENCE OF SITE SELECTION

Site selection is a multidisciplinary task that blends clinical access priorities with financial due diligence, legal research, and operational logistics. Successful behavioral health real estate teams begin with a wide funnel, identifying numerous candidate properties, then refine their options through progressive levels of analysis.

Key considerations include:

- Zoning compatibility and land use rights
- Accessibility for patients, staff, and emergency responders
- Environmental and infrastructure suitability
- Proximity to hospitals, social services, and transportation
- Risk exposure related to entitlement, community opposition, or site conditions

According to the Design-Build Institute of America (DBIA), over 60% of real estate project delays originate in the pre-development phase, largely due to overlooked zoning, permitting, or feasibility challenges.

SITE AND STRUCTURE DUE DILIGENCE FOR BUILDABILITY

Due diligence is not a box-checking exercise; it is a strategic investment in risk mitigation, budget control, and entitlement readiness. A rigorous due diligence process addresses both the physical characteristics of the land and the latent risks embedded in existing structures.

Best Practices in Site and Structure Due Diligence:

- Phase I and II Environmental Site Assessments: Identify contamination, hazardous materials, or historical land use conflicts.
- Soils and Geotechnical Reports: Evaluate grading needs, slope stability, soil bearing capacity, and foundation design viability.
- Utility Infrastructure Assessment: Confirm adequate water, sewer, gas, power, and telecom capacity, or quantify upgrade costs.
- Title Review and ALTA Surveys: Identify encumbrances, easements, and legal constraints that may restrict development.
- As-Built Building Evaluations (for adaptive reuse): Verify code compliance, structural integrity, HVAC lifespan, and energy performance.
- Civil Engineering Site Feasibility Reports: Provide early insight into stormwater management, drainage, and ADA grading solutions.
- Architectural Fit Studies and Programming Test Fits: Determine whether the clinical and operational program can be accommodated on the site.

Case Insight: A behavioral health developer in Orange County discovered unstable subsurface soils that would have added $600,000 in foundation mitigation costs. Early soil testing saved the client from closing on a site with hidden cost burdens.

KEY REAL ESTATE CRITERIA FOR BEHAVIORAL HEALTH FACILITIES

Accessibility:

Reaching Those Who Need Care Most Behavioral health facilities must be reachable by patients from all walks of life. Whether urban, suburban, or rural, access considerations include:

- Public transit stops within a quarter mile
- ADA-compliant sidewalks and entries
- Drop-off zones and well-lit, secure parking
- Geographic proximity to underserved populations. A San Francisco study showed behavioral clinics near major bus lines had a 30% lower no-show rate for appointments.

Zoning Laws:

Avoiding Regulatory Roadblocks Zoning and entitlement risks can delay projects for months or years. Success lies in:

- Early review of zoning ordinances and land use maps
- Identification of conditional use permit or variance requirements
- Pre-submittal meetings with planning departments
- Community engagement to avoid opposition-driven delays

Case Study: In Los Angeles County, early engagement by the Owner's Advisor helped secure a special use permit for a 16-bed mental health facility in a transitional neighborhood by addressing security and staffing plans transparently.

Proximity to Healthcare Networks Location decisions should enhance care coordination and reduce emergency department reliance:

- Close to hospitals, urgent care, and primary care providers
- Near housing services, detox centers, or job placement programs

- Within medical office or integrated healthcare zones

CONDUCTING A COMPREHENSIVE FEASIBILITY STUDY

Feasibility studies must move beyond surface metrics and into detailed risk and opportunity profiling. Components of a Robust Feasibility Study:

- Mental health market demand and service gap analysis
- Site fit studies for parking, programming, and access
- Preliminary project schedule, budget, and phasing plan
- Licensing and code pathway mapping (OSHPD, DHCS, ADA)
- Financial pro forma including land, construction, and operations. The Owner's Advisor must lead and coordinate this study with input from planners, architects, engineers, and clinical operators.

SUSTAINABILITY, COMMUNITY ALIGNMENT, AND LONG-TERM VIABILITY

A site is only as valuable as its long-term relevance. Sustainable behavioral health campuses:

- Incorporate energy-saving strategies and natural ventilation
- Include outdoor therapy gardens or patient courtyards
- Use landscaping that reinforces trauma-informed design
- Minimize operating costs through green building design

OVERCOMING BUREAUCRATIC AND COMMUNITY CHALLENGES

Winning Community Support:

- Host town halls with visual renderings and clear clinical plans
- Partner with neighborhood associations and schools

- Educate through data, testimonials, and site tours

Entitlement Acceleration Techniques:

- Engage local officials and planning staff before application
- Document neighborhood need for services and economic benefit
- Coordinate legal, political, and design narratives into a united front

Adaptive Reuse Opportunity: An underutilized post office in Alameda County was successfully converted into a behavioral health clinic after community forums, historic preservation consultation, and alignment with county mental health priorities.

CONCLUSION: SITE SELECTION AS A STRATEGIC INVESTMENT.NOT A GUESSING GAME

> "A successful project starts with a successful site, and a successful site is the result of deliberate, data-informed strategy."
>
> DATA SPECIALIST

Site selection is not a checkbox. It is the most consequential early decision in behavioral health real estate development. When mismanaged, poor site selection leads to downstream delays, budget overruns, licensure complications, and regulatory gridlock. When executed well with foresight, rigor, and collaboration, it becomes the foundation of a facility that heals, operates efficiently, and grows sustainably within its community.

THE HIGH COST OF POOR SITE SELECTION

Industry data confirms that up to 60% of real estate development delays can be traced back to challenges rooted in inadequate site analysis or poor due diligence (Design-Build Institute of America, 2022). Among the most common pitfalls:

- Zoning rejections or appeals that add 6-12 months to the entitlement schedule.
- Environmental or soil surprises (e.g., high water tables, hazardous materials) that require costly remediation.
- Utility service issues (inadequate water pressure, outdated infrastructure) that limit facility capacity or require design changes.
- Community opposition stemming from a lack of early engagement or poor site integration.

These are not rare edge cases; they are predictable and avoidable risks that strike behavioral health projects at a disproportionate rate due to their complexity and the stigmas often attached to mental health facilities.

DUE DILIGENCE: THE ESSENTIAL RISK MITIGATION TOOL

According to the American Institute of Architects (AIA), comprehensive due diligence in the site selection phase can reduce total project risk by up to 45%. That due diligence includes:

- ALTA surveys to identify encroachments, easements, and access limitations.
- Phase I and II Environmental Site Assessments (ESAs) to identify liabilities under Comprehensive Environmental Response, Compensation, and Liability Act (CERCLA).
- Geotechnical investigations to determine soil stability, seismic risk, and foundation requirements.
- Civil engineering assessments to evaluate stormwater, drainage, ADA pathways, grading, and floodplain compliance.
- Utility mapping and “will-serve” letters from water, sewer, power, telecom, and gas providers.
- Architectural fit studies to evaluate program compatibility with existing or proposed structures.

- Cost estimation and value engineering reviews to validate buildability, staging, and long-term O&M considerations.

Each of these processes uncovers risks, limitations, or hidden costs. Each is an opportunity to course-correct early, when the impact is minimal, instead of during construction, when change orders and delays are exponentially more expensive.

THE ROLE OF THE OWNER'S ADVISOR: MAXIMIZING INTELLIGENCE, MINIMIZING RISK

The most powerful advantage in the site selection and due diligence process is not a checklist; it's the expertise of the Owner's Advisor. As a subject matter expert across planning, permitting, behavioral health licensure, and facility delivery, the Owner's Advisor acts as:

- Risk anticipator: Identifying critical red flags during initial site screening.
- Process navigator: Coordinating with local planning departments, utility providers, and environmental consultants.
- Communications strategist: Building early support from stakeholders, civic leaders, and surrounding communities.
- Regulatory translator: Aligning zoning, code, and licensing requirements with the project's vision and constraints.

DBIA studies show that projects with strong early-stage Owner advisory leadership are 33% more likely to meet schedule targets, 26% more likely to stay within budget, and 56% less likely to experience litigation or agency conflict. These aren't theoretical gains; they are the difference between stalled and successful projects.

TRENDS DRIVING SMARTER SITE SELECTION

In today's climate of tight capital, labor shortages, and urgent demand for mental health services, site selection is increasingly driven by these evolving best practices:

- Proximity to underserved populations and data-driven identification of mental health care gaps (e.g., Health Professional Shortage Area (HPSA) and Substance Use Disorder (SUD) shortage areas).
- Adaptive reuse potential in vacant schools, offices, or retail centers offering cost and time savings of up to 40%.
- Transit-oriented development (TOD) to expand access and reduce transportation barriers for patients and staff.
- Environmental and social governance (ESG) metrics that favor sustainable site use and community-integrated designs.

The Owner's Advisor ensures that these drivers are not only considered, but translated into actionable site criteria and success metrics.

SUMMARY: BUILD ON CERTAINTY, NOT ASSUMPTIONS

Behavioral health real estate demands a foundation of clarity, not guesswork. That foundation begins with site selection, grounded in:

- Technical due diligence and risk identification
- Regulatory and zoning alignment
- Environmental and utility readiness
- Clinical and operational compatibility
- Community and stakeholder acceptance
- Financial feasibility and growth potential

When all of these factors are addressed proactively and in coordination with an experienced Owner's Advisor, the result is a site not just selected, but strategically secured.

FRONT LINE STORY # 10. MARKET ANALYSIS INSIGHT: UNCOVERING HIDDEN NEEDS

Our team was deep into a feasibility study for a new adult crisis stabilization unit (CSU). The county's official health plan pointed to a clear need, the funding seemed aligned, and all our preliminary work supported this direction. But something felt incomplete. The data we were using, while official, was nearly two years old, a lifetime in the world of public health.

Driven by a hunch, I started digging deeper, pulling raw data from local hospital emergency departments, school districts, and pediatricians. A startling pattern emerged: a dramatic, threefold increase in emergency psychiatric visits for adolescents over the past 18 months. This was a silent crisis, a wave of need that was building so fast it hadn't yet been reflected in the county's formal strategic plans. The system was focused on adults, but the most urgent, unaddressed need was for youth.

I brought the findings to our stakeholders. Pivoting the project was a significant risk. It meant re-evaluating our financial model, our architectural program, and our operational plan. But the data was undeniable. We made the call to shift our focus to an adolescent CSU. It was a challenging, complex pivot that required re-engaging our partners and making the case for a project that wasn't on anyone's official roadmap. Six months later, the county declared a pediatric mental health state of emergency, and our project was suddenly at the forefront of the solution. It was a powerful lesson in how market analysis is not just about confirming what we already know, but about uncovering the needs that no one is seeing yet.

FINAL THOUGHT

> "95% of a project's success is determined before the first brick is laid."
>
> DBIA CORE PRINCIPLES

That statement is truer in behavioral health than almost any other sector. The facility we dream of tomorrow (safe, dignified, healing, sustainable) must be born from the discipline and expertise we invest today.

With intelligent site selection, comprehensive due diligence, and an empowered Owner's Advisor at the helm, we don't just pick a property; we build a legacy of care.

Chapter 7

STAKEHOLDER Support and Public Partnership

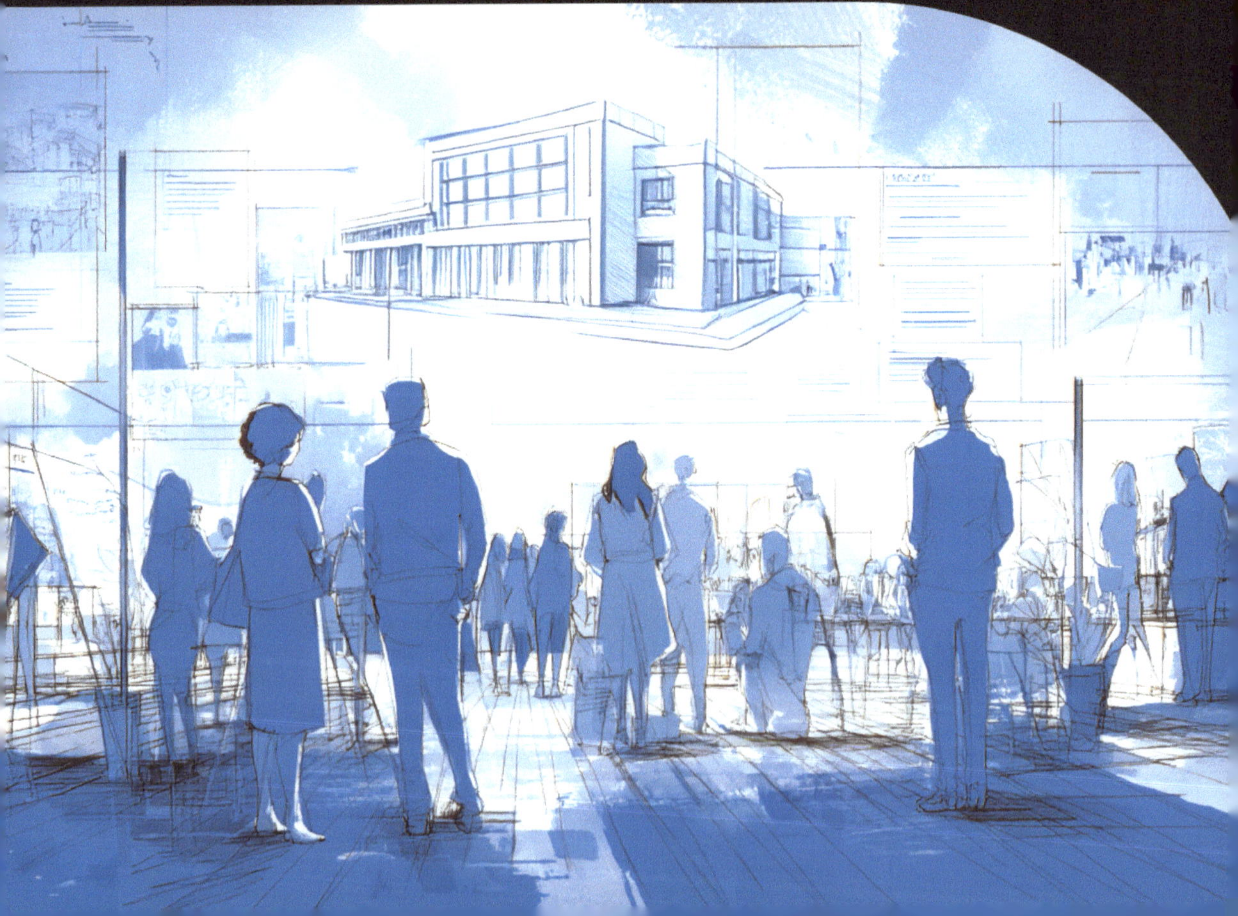

CHAPTER 7
STAKEHOLDER SUPPORT

WHAT YOU WILL LEARN IN THIS CHAPTER:

- Understanding Community Needs in Facility Planning and Development
- Building collaboration with stakeholders, community forums and advisory boards.
- Strategic Value of Building Stakeholder Support
- Examples of successful community partnerships in California
- Best Practices of Building Stakeholder Support

Pleasing personality, cooperation, and enthusiasm turn opposition into partnership. Lead with respect and steady presence. Behavioral health facilities succeed when teams listen, reflect, and show progress in public. Trust is built by making people feel heard and by doing what you said you would do.

Run stakeholder work as a core project stream. Map allies, neutrals, and opponents. Hold cadence meetings with clear notes and visible responses. Share design updates that show safety, dignity, and neighborhood fit. Keep a public-facing FAQ and update it as facts change.

FRONT LINE STORY# 11. BUILDING BRIDGES

> "The greatness of a community is most accurately measured by the compassionate actions of its members."
>
> CORETTA SCOTT KING

We were proposing a new transitional housing facility for young adults aging out of the foster care system, many of whom had significant behavioral health needs. The project was fully funded and desperately needed, but we faced a wall of opposition from the local homeowners' association. They held a community meeting filled with fear and misinformation, citing concerns about safety and property values. Our project was on the verge of being blocked before it even began.

Instead of fighting them in public hearings, we took a different approach. We identified the four most vocal opponents and invited them to a private meeting. We didn't bring charts or graphs. Instead, we brought two young people who had successfully transitioned out of a similar program in another city. For an hour, these two young adults shared their stories: their struggles with trauma and their dreams for the future. They didn't talk about real estate; they talked about their lives. One of the homeowners, a woman who had been our fiercest critic, began to cry. She said, "I never thought about who you were. I only thought about what you might do." By the end of the meeting, she had offered to organize a neighborhood welcome committee. We built a bridge not with data, but with dignity. That project was approved unanimously, and our most vocal opponents became our strongest advocates.

> "Stakeholders are not a barrier to progress -they are the path to success."
>
> DR. JUDITH RODIN, FORMER PRESIDENT OF THE ROCKEFELLER FOUNDATION

WHY STAKEHOLDER SUPPORT IS THE FOUNDATION OF EVERY SUCCESSFUL PROJECT

> "When it comes to building behavioral health facilities, the most important material isn't concrete—it's connection."
>
> OLD MAN RIVER

Behind every successful project is a network of support: local leaders who believe in the mission, residents who feel heard, healthcare systems eager to collaborate, and public agencies aligned on shared goals. **Stakeholder support isn't optional, it's essential.**

Enroll early and often with:

- Local neighbors and business owners
- City planning and zoning officials
- County behavioral health departments
- State licensing and funding agencies
- Adjacent hospitals and service providers
- Faith leaders, nonprofit organizers, and lived-experience advocates

Guiding principle: Work with the community, not around it.

FROM ENGAGEMENT TO ALIGNMENT: A PROVEN PATH

Stakeholder engagement is more than a checkbox, it's about **genuine relationships** built on shared goals and respect. Done well, it:

- Reduces resistance and **speeds approvals**
- Improves design relevance and **long-term performance**

California results (AIA, 2022):

- 2× more likely to meet long-term performance goals
- 1.5× more likely to stay on budget and schedule

Strategic benefits (DBIA, 2022):

- 23% faster entitlement approvals
- 35% fewer change orders
- 40% higher success meeting clinical/program goals

BEST PRACTICES FOR BUILDING STAKEHOLDER SUPPORT

1) Start Early

Begin outreach at concept, well before permit submissions or final design.

2) Create a Stakeholder Map

Identify key participants at every level:

- **Local:** neighborhood groups, nearby businesses, residents
- **City:** planning staff, councilmembers, permitting authorities
- **County/State:** BH agencies, housing, licensing
- **Clinical:** nearby hospitals, providers, case managers
- Use the map as your **momentum blueprint**.

3) Hold Community Forums & Listening Sessions

Invite input, surface concerns, and be transparent. Listening builds ownership.

4) Form an Advisory Board

Include clinicians, advocates, neighbors, and elected officials. Keep them engaged through **design, planning, and implementation**.

5) Partner with Local Champions

Leverage trusted leaders to open doors and build bridges across the community.

REAL-WORLD EXAMPLE: COLLABORATION IN ACTION

Facing early opposition to a 60-bed facility, a California team **paused to engage**:

- Hosted roundtables in churches and community centers
- Walked the neighborhood with local leaders
- Revised design (walking paths, gardens, security features) based on feedback

Outcome: Approval secured; the facility is now a **community-aligned model**, with former opponents as proud neighbors.

THE KEY TO SUCCESS: SHARED OWNERSHIP

Stakeholder support is a philosophy: Your voice matters.

In a complex field with compliance, funding, design, care, **aligned stakeholders** make everything easier.

UNDERSTANDING COMMUNITY NEEDS IN FACILITY PLANNING & DEVELOPMENT

CONDUCTING A COMPREHENSIVE COMMUNITY NEEDS ASSESSMENT

Stakeholder-informed planning starts with **data-driven assessment** to match facilities to local demand.

Key strategies

- Use public health data, census trends, ER utilization
- Engage diverse stakeholders: clinicians, leaders, patients, advocates
- Map existing services and identify care gaps
- Surface barriers: language, transportation, stigma, culture

1.1 How to Understand & Address Community Needs

Data collection: surveys, focus groups, interviews; supplement with public health and census data.

Identify gaps: crisis services, SUD treatment, youth/older adult services.

Address barriers: stigma, access, affordability, cultural competency.

Engage lived experience: include caregivers, peer leaders, service organizations, and local government.

1.2 Utilize Existing Data Sources

- State/county public health reports
- Hospital & ER utilization data
- Academic research and sector studies (e.g., SAMHSA; AIA Design & Health)

Blend new and existing data to target programming and service delivery.

INVOLVING THE COMMUNITY IN THE FACILITY DESIGN PROCESS

2.1 Participatory Design Strategies

Invite community input on:

- **Site selection:** accessibility, safety, neighborhood impact

- **Architectural features:** therapeutic, welcoming, not institutional
- **Program mix:** crisis stabilization, SUD treatment, family counseling, etc.

2.2 Host Community Workshops & Forums

Best practices

- **Design charrettes:** co-create layout and flow
- **Q&A forums:** address concerns openly with developers and clinicians
- **Digital engagement:** online surveys, virtual meetings, regular updates

STRENGTHENING TRUST & OWNERSHIP

3.1 Build Trust Through Transparency

- **Clear communication:** newsletters, town halls, social media
- **Proactive problem-solving:** safety, traffic, funding concerns handled collaboratively
- **Show the impact:** demonstrate how feedback informs design and operations

3.2 Empower Community Leadership

- **Advisory boards:** residents, patients, advocates as ongoing advisors
- **Volunteer & training programs:** equip locals to support operations
- **Public recognition:** celebrate contributions and milestones

MEASURING THE IMPACT OF COMMUNITY ENGAGEMENT

4.1 Establish Success Metrics

- **Participation levels:** workshop attendance, surveys, meetings

- **Design/service influence:** documented changes from feedback
- **Community satisfaction:** post-opening acceptance and impact

4.2 Commit to Continuous Improvement

- **Annual community check-ins** to inform adjustments
- **Ongoing advisory committees** for operational input
- **Share success stories** via testimonials and impact reports

Bottom line: Thoughtful, consistent engagement turns projects into **shared community assets** - easier to entitle, better to operate, and more effective in healing.

BUILDING COLLABORATION WITH STAKEHOLDERS, COMMUNITY FORUMS, AND ADVISORY BOARDS

Creating a successful behavioral health facility requires a broad coalition of support. Engage stakeholders early and often to build ownership and long-term alignment.

1) EARLY IDENTIFICATION OF KEY STAKEHOLDERS

Prioritize individuals and organizations with influence, insight, and local credibility.

Core groups include:

- **Community Members:** Future patients, caregivers, neighborhood leaders, and lived-experience advocates.
- **Local Organizations:** Nonprofits, faith groups, and advocacy organizations that offer insight and outreach.
- **Government Agencies:** Public health departments, zoning boards, funding and licensing authorities that can accelerate approvals.

- **Healthcare Providers:** Hospitals, clinics, and behavioral health professionals who ensure integrated care pathways.
- **Law Enforcement and First Responders:** Critical partners for crisis response and safety planning.

2) ENGAGEMENT TECHNIQUES THAT BUILD TRUST

- Community workshops and design charrettes
- Advisory boards with lived-experience representation
- Transparent Q&A forums
- Online surveys, bilingual resources, and social media outreach

3) FORMALIZING PARTNERSHIPS

- Use Memorandums of Understanding to define roles and responsibilities
- Create community benefit agreements where appropriate
- Align engagement milestones with development phases and decision gates

THE STRATEGIC VALUE OF STAKEHOLDER ENGAGEMENT

Stakeholder engagement is not a checkbox. It builds shared ownership that supports operational success, political resilience, and community integration. When people help shape the process, the facility reflects local needs, values, and identity.

KEY BENEFITS OF COMPREHENSIVE STAKEHOLDER ENGAGEMENT

- Reduces NIMBY opposition through education, transparency, and trust building
- Accelerates entitlements and permitting by securing city and county support early

- Improves facility design and functionality through local and clinical input
- Secures long-term funding and partnerships through civic and political alignment
- Enhances safety and social acceptance, reducing stigma and increasing utilization
- Builds advocacy networks that endure beyond ribbon cutting

EXAMPLES OF SUCCESSFUL COMMUNITY PARTNERSHIPS IN CALIFORNIA

✅ 1. San Diego Behavioral Health Hub

Resident-led planning sessions influenced the therapeutic layout, inclusion of outdoor spaces, and culturally relevant programs.

This references the San Diego County Behavioral Health Services Community-Based Continuum of Care, including projects like the new Behavioral Health Hub in Hillcrest (as part of the UC San Diego redevelopment) and community-informed behavioral health planning through the Behavioral Health Advisory Board (BHAB). Public Engagement: San Diego County uses stakeholder sessions and resident feedback to guide service delivery and site selection.

📚 Source: San Diego County BHS Strategic Plan

✅ 2. Sacramento Crisis Stabilization Unit

Partnership with law enforcement and community mental health nonprofits reduced ER overflows and improved referral coordination.

The Sacramento County Mental Health Treatment Center includes a Crisis Stabilization Unit (CSU) developed in partnership with the county, community health providers, and local law enforcement to reduce ER visits and improve psychiatric crisis response.

📚 Source: Sacramento County Health Services

☑️ **3. Los Angeles County Youth Mental Health Initiative**

Youth advisory boards helped shape engagement strategy, branding, and peer support design.

LA County launched the Youth Mental Health Initiative as part of the Mental Health Services Act (MHSA) programming. The program used Youth Advisory Boards, peer support, and direct youth engagement in service design. Example: The WeRise LA program and youth-focused mental health coalitions help guide service design and communications.

📚 Source: LA County Department of Mental Health

Each of these projects demonstrates the transformative impact of participatory development -achieving faster approvals, better utilization, and deeper community buy-in.

BEST PRACTICES FOR BUILDING STAKEHOLDER SUPPORT

1) START EARLY, STAY ENGAGED

Stakeholder engagement is most effective when it begins in pre-development and continues through occupancy.

2) MAP STAKEHOLDER GROUPS INTELLIGENTLY

- Include vulnerable and underrepresented populations
- Coordinate messaging with public health agencies
- Train team members in cultural competency and trauma-informed communication

3) CREATE FEEDBACK LOOPS

- Track how community input informs design decisions

- Provide formal updates and "you said, we did" reports
- Celebrate local contributions and milestones in public forums

4) MEASURE ENGAGEMENT OUTCOMES

- Number of participants and events
- Design or policy changes linked to public input
- Post-occupancy satisfaction and utilization metrics

5) COLLABORATE WITH A SKILLED OWNER'S ADVISOR

A strategic Owner's Advisor can:

- Translate community input into actionable development strategies
- Facilitate stakeholder workshops
- Align public engagement with entitlement and funding goals

CONCLUSION: STAKEHOLDER SUPPORT AS THE CORNERSTONE OF SUSTAINABLE BEHAVIORAL HEALTH DEVELOPMENT

Behavioral health real estate development does not occur in a vacuum; it unfolds in real neighborhoods, on real streets, among real people with opinions, concerns, and hopes. Success depends not only on permits, funding, and design, but also on the willing participation of a diverse network of stakeholders.

Stakeholder support is not a "nice to have"; it is a core requirement for long-term success. The data is clear:

- Projects with integrated stakeholder planning are up to **35%** more likely to meet budget and schedule targets
- Facilities co-designed with local users report **38%** higher early engagement and **50%** better alignment with program goals

- For every **$1** invested in early community engagement, developers save about **$4** in reduced conflicts and delays (World Bank, 2020)

Facilities built **with** communities, not only **for** them, are safer, better utilized, and more resilient to political and operational challenges. When community voices shape design, programming, and operations, the result becomes more than a project; it becomes a legacy.

BUILDING A LEGACY, NOT JUST A BUILDING

Stakeholder engagement is not a line item; it is the glue that binds design to dignity, funding to function, and operations to outcomes. When we build with community, we create facilities that are not only physically sustainable but also socially, politically, and economically resilient. These projects become neighborhood cornerstones, sources of healing and pride, and they endure.

DBIA findings for projects that structure community engagement from the start:

- **35%** fewer post-construction change orders
- **23%** higher on-time delivery rates
- Higher community utilization and satisfaction scores

Done well, stakeholder engagement mitigates risk, secures faster entitlements, builds goodwill with agencies, and lifts facility success across the board. It also equips the Owner's Advisor to build trust, translate concerns into solutions, and align development goals with local realities.

As we continue through the Wellspring Manual, we will build on this foundation: facility programming, therapeutic design, and construction management best practices. It all starts here, with people, trust, measurable participation, and the courage to engage deeply, honestly, and inclusively.

Chapter 8

Facility **PROGRAMMING** and Conceptual Design

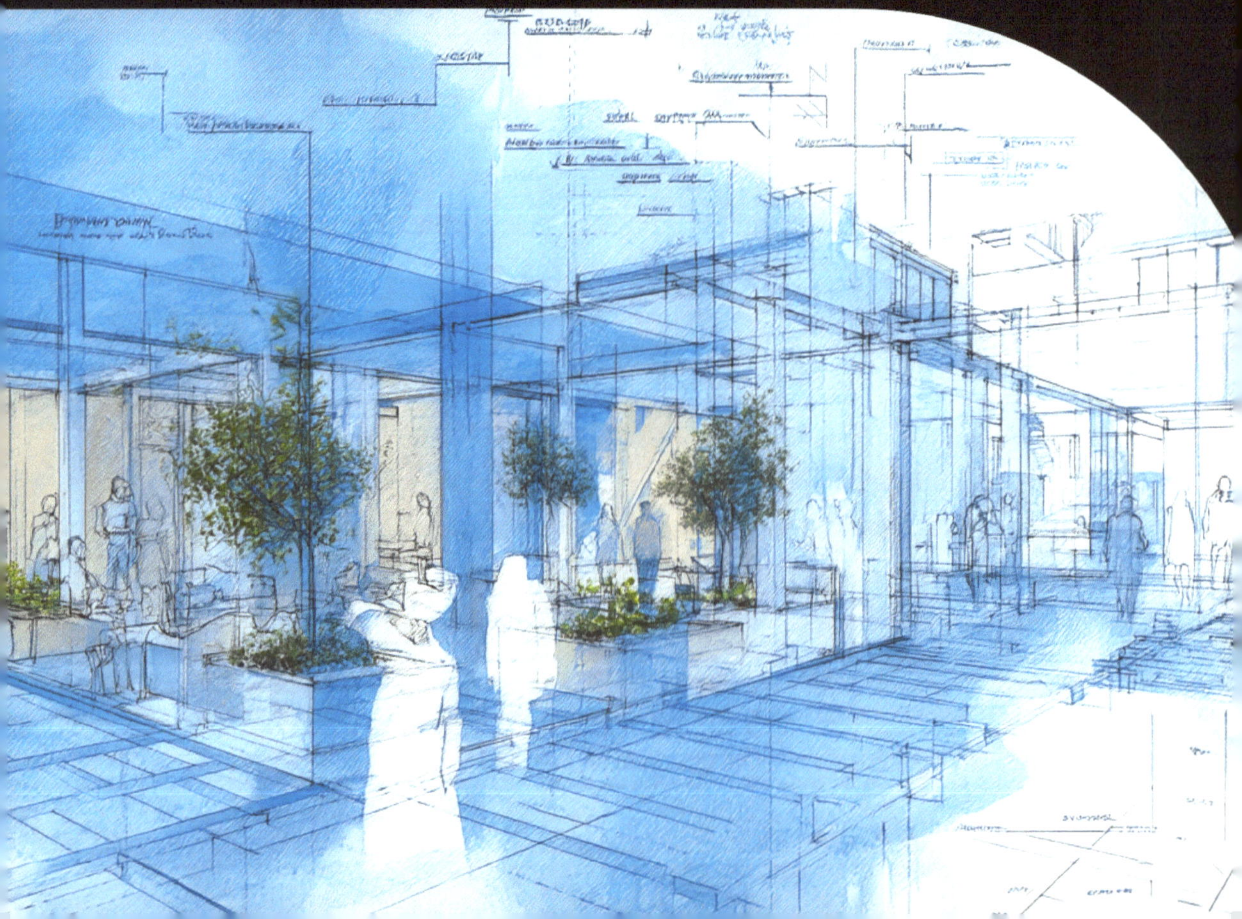

CHAPTER 8
FACILITY PROGRAMMING AND CONCEPTUAL DESIGN

WHAT YOU WILL LEARN IN THIS CHAPTER:

- Aligning Clinical Needs with Built Environments
- Space Planning for Trauma-Informed Care and Safety
- Integrated Care Models and Functional Adjacencies
- Early Cost Modeling and Phasing Strategies

Imagination translates care models into rooms, flows, and moments that heal. Creative vision must stay anchored in therapeutic needs. In behavioral health, programming is how dignity, safety, and outcomes become floor area and adjacencies.

Turn vision into program requirements the team can cost and build. Facilitate workshops with clinicians and operations. Write clear Room Data Sheets. Create test fits to validate flows for intake, de-escalation, staff respite, and family visits. Price options so choices can be made quickly.

ENGAGING STAKEHOLDERS IN THE DESIGN VISION

Programming and conceptual design form the foundation of successful behavioral health real estate development. At this critical stage, strategic vision is translated into the built environment, shaping not only the operational flow of care but the very experience of healing. The environments we create for behavioral health care are more than spaces; they are therapeutic ecosystems. These settings must be safe, trauma-informed, adaptable, inclusive, sustainable, and technologically integrated. Every room, every corridor, and every design decision carries the potential to advance or hinder a patient's recovery, a clinician's effectiveness, and an organization's mission. This chapter explores how to align behavioral health, medical, and clinical needs with space programming, integrate care delivery models into design, use early cost modeling to inform decisions, and ensure that every stakeholder (patients, providers, funders, and regulators) is engaged in shaping facilities built for lasting impact.

ALIGNING CLINICAL NEEDS WITH BUILT ENVIRONMENTS

TRANSLATING SERVICES INTO FUNCTIONAL SPACE

Behavioral health facilities must support specific populations and care modalities such as crisis stabilization, outpatient therapy, residential treatment, and intensive care. Each model requires spaces that:

- Accommodate clinical interventions such as therapy, medication administration, and diagnostics
- Enable 24/7 staff supervision and collaboration
- Ensure patient safety and privacy
- Support transitions between care levels such as triage to stabilization

CLINICAL STAFF AS DESIGN PARTNERS

Programming begins with dialogue. Engage staff through interviews, workflow shadowing, and design validation workshops to surface:

- Preferred room adjacencies
- Critical supervision and security needs
- Optimal circulation and flow
- Equipment, information technology, and accessibility priorities

REGULATORY AND LICENSING ALIGNMENT

Design must meet the standards of:

- State licensing authorities
- The Joint Commission
- CMS and Medi-Cal, as applicable
- NFPA Life Safety Code
- Facilities Guidelines Institute Behavioral Health Design Guidelines

SPACE PLANNING FOR TRAUMA-INFORMED CARE AND SAFETY

Principles of Trauma-Informed Design

- **Safety:** Visual clarity, ligature resistance, and emergency preparedness
- **Empowerment:** Autonomy-supportive features such as lighting control and privacy options
- **Calmness:** Reduced noise, soft color palettes, and biophilic elements
- **Trust:** Non-institutional, welcoming environments with appropriate staff visibility

Design Strategies

- Unobstructed lines of sight to enable passive supervision
- Soft seating, warm lighting, and natural textures
- Access to nature through views and outdoor areas
- Anti-ligature fixtures and tamper-resistant materials
- Multipurpose rooms that adapt to evolving care needs

CASE EXAMPLE: SANTA CLARA COUNTY BEHAVIORAL HEALTH

By integrating daylight, healing gardens, and trauma-informed interior finishes, the Santa Clara facility reported more than a 20 percent reduction in staff stress and patient incidents according to post-occupancy surveys.

FRONT LINE STORY # 12. DESIGN INNOVATION

> "Design is not just what it looks like and feels like. Design is how it works."
>
> STEVE JOBS

We were designing a crisis stabilization unit for a county that had seen a sharp rise in patients presenting with extreme agitation and sensory overload. The standard clinical model called for small, isolated seclusion rooms for de-escalation. But our clinical team challenged us to think differently, arguing that traditional seclusion can feel punitive and re-traumatizing. They asked, "How can the environment itself be a tool for calming?"

This question led to a design innovation: the 'sensory modulation room.' Working with occupational therapists and acoustical engineers, we designed a small suite of rooms adjacent to the main triage area. Each room was outfitted with tools that allowed patients to self-regulate. One had weighted blankets, ambient sound machines, and aromatherapy diffusers. Another featured tactile walls with different textures and adjustable, dimmable lighting controls that cycled through calming colors. Instead of being placed in an empty room, patients could choose a space and actively engage in their own de-escalation. The innovation was a success.Post-occupancy data showed that the use of physical restraints dropped by over 40% in the first year.

This dramatic 40% reduction in restraint use demonstrates how thoughtful environmental design can directly improve patient outcomes and dignity in behavioral health settings. By treating the environment as a therapeutic tool, we enhanced patient dignity and created a safer space for everyone.

INTEGRATED CARE MODELS AND FUNCTIONAL ADJACENCIES

WHAT IS INTEGRATED BEHAVIORAL HEALTH?

Integrated behavioral health combines primary care, psychiatry, case management, and social services in one coordinated environment. Facility programming should support:

- Flexible clinical spaces for co-located teams
- Shared records and collaborative care plans
- Informal zones for impromptu consultation and case huddles

KEY SPATIAL RELATIONSHIPS

- Exam rooms located near therapy rooms
- Medication management adjacent to medical consults
- Observation areas directly linked to intake and triage
- Staff break rooms and respite zones separated from care delivery

Example: Los Angeles Mental Health Urgent Care Center

Integrated triage, medical clearance, and peer navigation zones are designed for same-day diversion from emergency departments. Functional adjacency planning reduced average intake to treatment time by 40 percent.

EARLY COST MODELING AND PHASING STRATEGIES

Estimating from the Start

Cost control begins in programming. Align early cost data with clinical goals to enable prioritization and phasing:

- Parametric estimating based on program square footage
- Elemental cost breakdowns per room and per system
- Target value design that designs to the budget rather than only estimating after design

Phased Implementation Models

- **Phase 1:** Emergency intake, triage, stabilization
- **Phase 2:** Outpatient services, counseling, family support
- **Phase 3:** Permanent supportive housing and community programs

Scalability by Design

- Future-ready floor plates
- Infrastructure stubs for expansion
- Demountable walls and plug-in technology zones

ENGAGING STAKEHOLDERS IN THE DESIGN VISION

Who to Engage

- Healthcare providers and facility users
- Patients and families, including advisory boards
- Funders, licensing officials, and Authorities Having Jurisdiction
- Community partners and advocacy groups

Engagement Strategies

- Interactive charrettes and journey mapping
- Mock-up room walk-throughs
- Visual preference surveys
- Decision logs and design narrative sign-offs

Example: San Diego Youth Behavioral Health Center

Stakeholder sessions identified the need for family waiting rooms, gender-sensitive restrooms, and distinct youth and adult therapy wings. Implementing these priorities strengthened community support and reduced rework.

FRONT LINE STORY# 13. STAKEHOLDER ENGAGEMENT

> "The only way to do great work is to love what you do."
>
> STEVE JOBS

During the conceptual design phase for a large behavioral health campus, we knew that engaging the frontline staff would be critical. These were the nurses, social workers, and mental health technicians who would live and breathe in this space every day. An architectural plan can look perfect on paper, but it's the staff who know the reality of patient flow, sightlines, and security needs.

We went beyond typical feedback sessions. We built full-scale mock-ups of key rooms.a patient room, a nurse's station, and a therapy office.out of cardboard and inexpensive furniture. Then, we invited the entire clinical and support staff to walk through the mock-ups and simulate their daily routines. The insights were immediate and invaluable. Nurses realized the proposed layout of their station created a critical blind spot. The maintenance crew pointed out that the placement of an access panel in a patient room was a security risk. A therapist noted that the desk orientation in the therapy office would feel confrontational to a patient. We documented every piece of feedback and used it to refine the final construction drawings. This deep level of stakeholder engagement didn't just prevent costly change orders; it fostered a profound sense of ownership and excitement among the staff. They weren't just being handed a new building; they were co-creating their future workplace.

CREATING THERAPEUTIC, SUSTAINABLE, AND TECHNOLOGY-INTEGRATED ENVIRONMENTS

KEY PRINCIPLES OF THERAPEUTIC ENVIRONMENTS

- **Safety first:** Ligature-resistant fixtures, panic buttons, secure access
- **Natural light:** Windows, skylights, circadian-friendly lighting systems
- **Calm aesthetics:** Non-glare surfaces, acoustic insulation, biophilic textures
- **Personalization:** Patient control in private areas where appropriate
- **Cultural competence:** Design that reflects community identity

CASE STUDIES IN BEHAVIORAL HEALTH FACILITY DESIGN

San Francisco Behavioral Health Center

- Achieved LEED Silver certification
- Integrated private patios and personalized patient zones

- Reported 18% improvement in staff retention within one year

East LA Wellness Hub

- Co-designed with neighborhood leaders
- Included community art installations and multilingual signage
- Increased service utilization by 35% over projected levels

INTEGRATING TECHNOLOGY

- **Telehealth zones:** Private, acoustically treated kiosks
- **Smart building systems:** Automated lighting, HVAC, and patient comfort controls
- **Patient monitoring:** Non-invasive observation technology linked to nurse stations
- **Data dashboards:** Real-time occupancy and scheduling systems

SUSTAINABILITY AND RESILIENCE

- **Energy efficiency:** Passive solar, daylighting, zoned HVAC
- **Water conservation:** Low-flow plumbing, rain capture, greywater reuse where permissible
    - Regulations vary by state and municipality
    - Practical applications include routing washing machine drainage to indoor or outdoor gardens
- **Emergency preparedness:** Backup power, seismic upgrades, fireproofing

Example: Sacramento Behavioral Health Hub

- Reduced energy consumption by 30% using high-performance windows, thermal mass strategies, and solar PV arrays
- Qualified for long-term operating subsidies

CONCLUSION: DESIGNING WITH PURPOSE, HEALING WITH INTENTION

Programming and conceptual design are more than early milestones in a project; they are the soul-setting moments where mission becomes form, and form becomes function. In behavioral health real estate, these early decisions echo through every phase of development, construction, and operation. They shape not just walls and workflows, but the very culture of care. At this foundational stage, clarity of purpose is paramount. Facilities must be designed not only to meet licensing requirements or code compliance but to actively support clinical excellence, patient dignity, and operational efficiency. They must be safe yet non-institutional, calming yet clinically robust, flexible yet carefully choreographed for security, supervision, and service delivery.

BEST PRACTICES IN BEHAVIORAL HEALTH DESIGN PROGRAMMING

1. **Lead with clinical intent**
   - Anchor programming in the care strategy. Whether crisis stabilization, long-term recovery, or outpatient care, align spaces with therapeutic models and pathways from day one.
2. **Design for trauma-informed healing**
   - Select materials, lighting, acoustics, privacy measures, and user controls that reduce anxiety, support autonomy, and create emotional safety for patients, staff, and families.
3. **Support integrated care models**
   - Place care team areas and service lines to optimize functional adjacencies, reduce transfer stress, and enable collaborative workflows.
4. **Plan with phasing in mind**
   - Incorporate modular options, shelled space, and staged activations to accommodate growth, flexibility, and evolving service needs.

5. **Utilize early cost modeling**
   - Align scope with budget using cost-informed programming and preconstruction collaboration. Begin value engineering at concept, not after bids.
6. **Engage multidisciplinary stakeholders**
   - Include voices from every level: clinicians, frontline staff, peer advocates, maintenance teams, and patients. Design for all layers of experience.
7. **Avoid late reprogramming**
   - Do not rush or skip clinical input. Validate space needs with mock-ups, test fits, and real-world walkthroughs to prevent costly redesigns.
8. **Balance innovation with licensing reality**
   - Harmonize vision with DHCS, HCAI, ADA, and local fire and life safety requirements.
9. **Clarify roles in early design coordination**
   - Assign responsibility for decisions, document control, and design verification across architect, Owner's Advisor, and clinical leadership.
10. **Plan for operational transitions**
    - Design for opening day and for Day 100 and Day 365. Address maintenance, patient flow, infection control, and staff efficiency from the start.

DESIGN AS A BRIDGE BETWEEN STRATEGY AND EXPERIENCE

At its best, behavioral health facility design is not about architecture for its own sake; it is about outcomes. The right layout reduces aggression. The right light improves sleep. The right materials support de-escalation. The right adjacencies reduce staff fatigue. Design becomes medicine, and the facility becomes a silent partner in the healing process.

When vision is translated into programming with clarity and discipline, behavioral health buildings become more than places; they become instruments of care. They become environments that elevate clinical performance, reduce stigma, and invite communities to see mental health treatment not as a last resort, but as a natural and compassionate part of wellness.

As we move forward in the Wellspring Manual, we'll build on this design foundation, exploring how programming becomes construction, how staffing meets space, and how clinical outcomes are shaped from every architectural detail. But it all begins here: with thoughtful planning, engaged collaboration, and a commitment to design that heals.

> "A building is not just a container. It is a teacher, a tool, a mirror, and if done right, a source of hope."
>
> BRIAN JONES

Chapter 9

DESIGN Best Practices for Behavioral Health Facilities

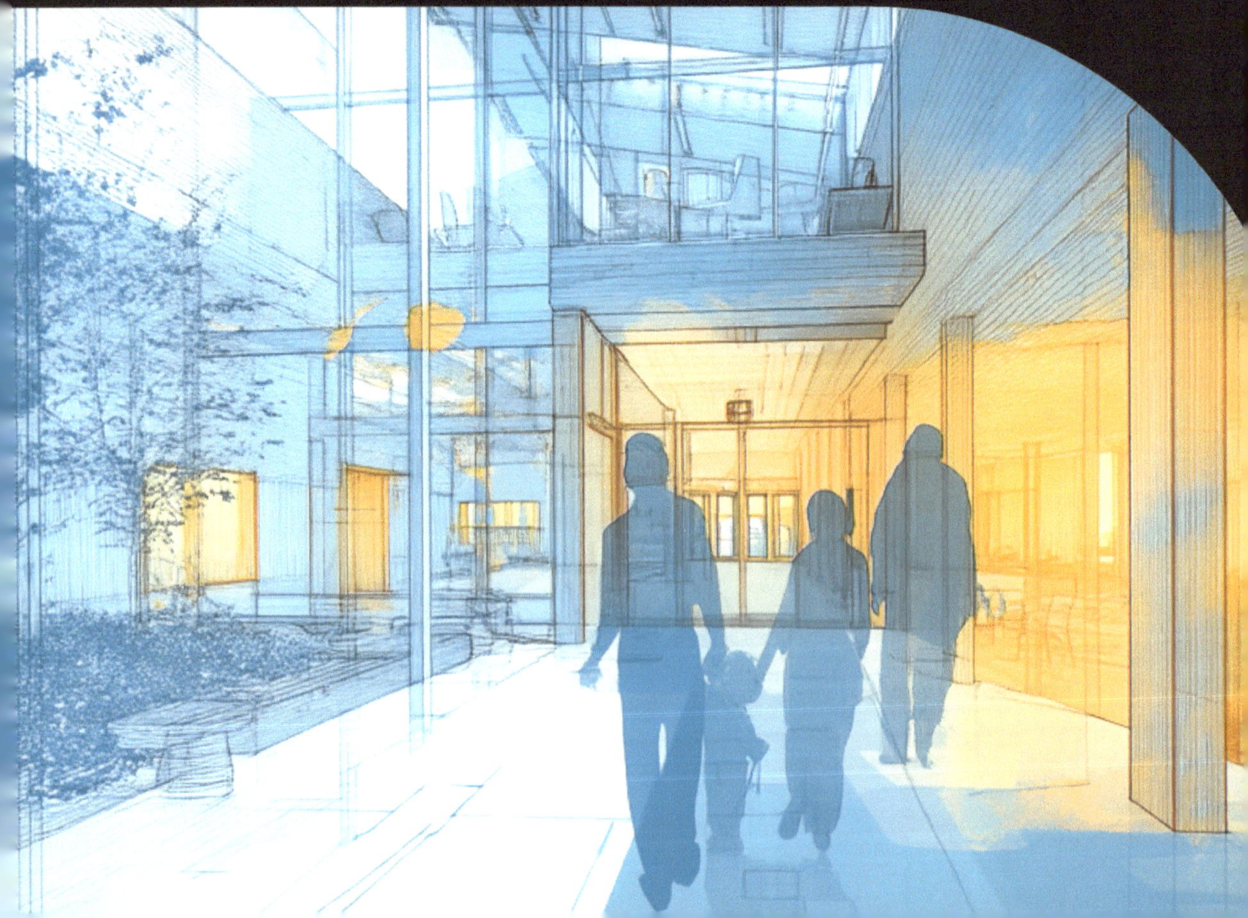

CHAPTER 9
BEST PRACTICES FOR BEHAVIORAL HEALTH CARE DESIGN

"If you think good design is expensive, you should look at the cost of bad design."

DR. RALF SPETH

WHAT YOU WILL LEARN IN THIS CHAPTER

- **Best Practices for Behavioral Health Care Facility Design**
- **The Big Five Best Practices**
- **Top 100 Best Practices for Behavioral Health Design**
- **Design Documentation Best Practices for Complex Systems**
- **Coordination Between Disciplines for Constructability**
- **Infection Control, Security, Ligature Resistance, and Accessibility**
- **Design for Healing, Treatment, and Recovery**
- **Managing Evolving User Needs Without Compromising Schedule**
- **Owner Review Cycles and Document Control Protocols**

CHAPTER OVERVIEW

Design Development is where vision meets precision. It is the technical phase where conceptual layouts evolve into construction-ready documents. In behavioral health real estate, this step is mission-critical. Behavioral health facilities involve sensitive populations, highly regulated care environments, and layered interdisciplinary needs. As such, design must be purposeful, clinically aligned, code-compliant, cost-aware, and fully coordinated.

This chapter is structured around six essential components of facility design, with a focus on The BIG 5 and The 100 Best Practices of Design and risk mitigation strategies for real estate professionals, developers, owner's advisors, architects, and clinical operators.

Organized planning and imagination meet in design. Protect dignity and safety without institutionalizing the experience. Behavioral health facilities deserve spaces that calm, orient, and restore.

Translate intent into standards and details the field can build. Use evidence-based checklists for ligature resistance, wayfinding, acoustics, and daylight. Run constructability reviews early. Pair mockups with user walkthroughs so feedback improves documents before hard costs lock. Apply trauma-informed principles consistently.

> "Architecture should speak of its time and place, but yearn for timelessness."
>
> FRANK GEHRY

FRONT LINE STORY #14. DESIGN FOR HEALING

A residential treatment center we were renovating had chronic issues with patient agitation, particularly in the evenings. The facility was older, with long, narrow corridors lit by harsh fluorescent lights. During the renovation, our team focused on biophilic and trauma-informed design. We replaced the institutional lighting with a tunable, circadian rhythm system that produced warmer, dimmer light in the evenings. We widened a key corridor to create a small, open seating area with a view of a newly planted garden. We also installed acoustic panels to dampen noise.

The post-occupancy data was striking. Evening agitation incidents dropped by over 30%, and the use of PRN (as-needed) anxiety medication decreased significantly. It was a powerful demonstration that the building itself could be a therapeutic intervention. The environment wasn't just a container for care; it was an active part of the healing process.

THE IMPACT OF DESIGN EXCELLENCE IN BEHAVIORAL HEALTH

Why it matters

Design shapes how patients heal, how staff perform, and how systems function. In behavioral health settings, high quality and well coordinated design elevates safety, dignity, operational efficiency, cost control, and long term community impact.

EVIDENCE HIGHLIGHTS

Research from the Center for Health Design and the American Institute of Architects shows that evidence based design in behavioral health facilities is associated with:

- **30–50%** improvement in patient satisfaction and overall experience
- **20–25%** reduction in aggressive behaviors and use of restraints
- **15–18%** decrease in elopement and self harm incidents
- Up to **40%** improvement in staff retention and job satisfaction

According to the Design Build Institute of America 2023 Benchmarking Report, projects that apply strategic design coordination early:

- Are **43%** more likely to finish on time and under budget

- See **50%** fewer change orders during construction
- Achieve faster licensing approval and operational readiness

WHAT MAKES DESIGN EFFECTIVE

Healing centered design blends architecture, behavioral science, clinical insight, and community engagement to:

- Improve safety and reduce operational risk
- Lower lifecycle costs and support budget discipline
- Increase program flexibility and future adaptability
- Build trust and pride among staff, patients, and families

WHAT THIS CHAPTER COVERS

- The **Top 100 Best Practices** in behavioral health design
- Trauma informed principles and biophilic strategies
- Adaptable layouts and constructability that is affordable and durable
- How early involvement of experienced design teams and Owner's Advisors produces environments that are clinically responsive, financially sustainable, and socially meaningful

THE BIG 5 BEST PRACTICES FOR BEHAVIORAL HEALTH DESIGN EXCELLENCE

Designing for behavioral health care is not simply about meeting codes or achieving operational efficiency. It is about creating dignified, therapeutic environments that uplift, heal, and empower. Environments directly affect clinical outcomes, staff well-being, patient recovery, and long-term operational sustainability. According to the American Institute of Architects (AIA) and the Center for Health Design (CHD), behavioral health facilities designed with evidence-based strategies report 30-50% higher patient satisfaction, lower incidents of aggression, and improved staff retention.

Here are the foundational cornerstones, The Big 5 Best Practices, that must guide every behavioral health facility's architectural journey:

1. Trauma-Informed and Neurologically Attuned Design: Design environments that minimize cognitive overload, prioritize emotional regulation, and promote safety. Individuals in behavioral health treatment often experience heightened sensitivity to noise, light, and unpredictability. Trauma-informed design incorporates soft finishes, muted color palettes, and simple layouts that reduce stress and foster control. Research shows a 34% reduction in agitation-related incidents and a 22% decrease in restraint use in trauma-informed spaces (CHD, 2022).

2. Biophilic Design: Reconnect patients and staff with natural systems through daylight, green views, organic textures, and environmental rhythms. Access to daylight has been shown to reduce depression symptoms by 30% and accelerate patient recovery by 15-20% (Ulrich, 1984; Terrapin Bright Green, 2021). Biophilic spaces lower cortisol levels, promote circadian rhythm alignment, and increase staff alertness and satisfaction.

3. Outdoor Therapeutic Spaces: Healing gardens, enclosed courtyards, patios for group therapy, and nature-based programming create immersive recovery experiences. According to the University of Washington's Department of Psychiatry (2021), facilities incorporating outdoor therapeutic zones report a 17% drop in medication reliance and 20% higher patient engagement rates. These spaces support movement, reduce agitation, and offer calming escape routes for de-escalation.

4. Flexible Layouts and Universal Design: Design for adaptability; program spaces to evolve with changing care models, census levels, or regulatory needs. Using universal room types, demountable walls, and infrastructure for future services (e.g., shelled space) ensures capital efficiency. The AIA's 2022 Design for Adaptability report found that flexible design reduces renovation costs by up to 40% over a facility's life cycle and improves readiness for integrated behavioral health models.

5. Strategic Design: Leadership and Owner's Advisor Oversight Early involvement of an Owner's Advisor, paired with healthcare-specialized architects, ensures that every design decision supports the facility's clinical mission, funding strategy, and long-term sustainability. According to the 2023 DBIA Benchmarking Report, projects with an Owner's Advisor involved from pre-design are 43% more likely to be delivered on time and under budget, with 50% fewer change orders and significantly smoother licensing outcomes. These leaders align technical details with operational realities.

Together, these BIG 5 best practices form the bedrock of high-performing, human-centered behavioral health architecture. The spaces we build speak not only to function, but to dignity, hope, and transformation. The rest of this chapter builds upon these principles to outline the top 100 design best practices shaping the future of behavioral health care.

THE OWNER'S ADVISOR: GUARDIAN OF ALIGNMENT AND DELIVERY

The Owner's Advisor Ensures:

- **Licensure, mission, and clinical model alignment**
- **Schedule and scope clarity** throughout design
- **Real-time feedback integration** from operators and funders

Projects with full Owner's Advisor involvement during design are **43% more likely** to finish on time and under budget, and experience **50% fewer redesign delays** (DBIA, 2023).

BUILDING A BRIGHTER FUTURE THROUGH DESIGN

Design is **policy in built form** -it shapes dignity, hope, and care in ways people can touch and feel. With **research-backed strategies** and **cross-functional collaboration**, behavioral health facilities can become places that truly heal.

Priorities for Behavioral Health Design:

- **Patient-Centered** – Every choice grounded in safety, dignity, and healing
- **Nature-Connected** – Environments that integrate natural light, views, and restorative landscapes
- **Future-Adaptable** – Flexible spaces prepared for evolving models of care
- **Collaboratively Crafted** – Shaped through inclusive teamwork across disciplines

FRONT LINE STORY #15. MANAGING CHANGE

> "The only constant in life is change."
>
> HERACLITUS

Halfway through the design development for a new outpatient clinic, the county received a new grant to co-locate a small pharmacy and lab services within the facility. This was a major programmatic shift that threatened to derail our schedule. Instead of starting the design over, we used a "surgical" approach.

We had intentionally designed the clinic with a modular grid and universal room sizes. Working with the architect, we identified a block of four adjacent therapy offices that could be converted. Because the core plumbing and electrical infrastructure was already planned to be robust in that zone, we were able to re-program the space for the pharmacy and lab with minimal changes to the main building shell and systems. This flexible, forward-thinking design allowed us to accommodate a major change with only a three-week impact on the schedule, saving the project from a months-long delay and ensuring the community received these vital new services.

TOP 100 BEST PRACTICES FOR BEHAVIORAL HEALTH CARE DESIGN

> "When you change the design of a space, you change the experience of the people who enter it."

DR. EVE EDELSTEIN, NEURO-ARCHITECT

The following **100 best practices for BH Design** integrate the most current research, thought leadership, and proven strategies in architecture, planning, and healthcare design. They are intended to inspire and guide the finest formulations in behavioral health facility development.

1. **Trauma-Informed and Neurologically Attuned Design** – Support cognitive and emotional stability by minimizing sensory overload and environmental triggers.
2. **Biophilic Design** – Integrate natural elements like light, greenery, and organic forms to promote psychological recovery.
3. **Outdoor Therapeutic Spaces** – Walking paths, gardens, and shaded gathering areas decrease anxiety and foster social connection.
4. **Flexible Layouts and Modular Design** – Enable adaptability through modular rooms and partitions.
5. **Strategic Design Leadership and Owner's Advisor Oversight** – Engage advisors early to align budget, schedule, and design integrity.
6. **Abundant Natural Light** – Daylight in patient areas shortens hospital stays and improves mood.
7. **Green Views and Exterior Vistas** – Provide sightlines to greenery to reduce stress and aggression.
8. **Acoustic Comfort and Sound Dampening** – Lower noise to improve concentration and reduce agitation.
9. **Non-Institutional Aesthetic** – Use residential-like touches to reduce stigma and increase satisfaction.
10. **Patient-Controlled Environments** – Give patients control over light, temperature, and sensory input.
11. **Post-Occupancy Evaluations (POEs)** – Measure outcomes at 6 and 12 months to refine design.
12. **Sensory Integration Zones** – Multisensory rooms for grounding and emotional regulation.

13. **Cultural and Community Representation** – Reflect cultural relevance to increase trust and access.
14. **Safety Through Visibility and Passive Observation** – Maintain supervision without intrusive surveillance.
15. **Gender-Inclusive and Identity-Affirming Design** – Support privacy and dignity for all identities.
16. **Wayfinding and Orientation Design** – Use intuitive layouts, symbols, and color cues.
17. **Calming Zones for De-Escalation** – Provide sensory modulation rooms to reduce restraints.
18. **Staff Zones that Promote Wellness** – Include break and reflection spaces to reduce burnout.
19. **Family Engagement Areas** – Create supportive rooms for family involvement in care.
20. **Compact and Intuitive Circulation Paths** – Simplify corridors to enhance safety and speed.
21. **Accessible and Ergonomic Workstations** – Inclusive nurse stations that reduce staff injury.
22. **Hands-Free Fixtures** – Motion-activated systems to improve hygiene.
23. **Smart Facility Systems** – IoT for air quality, occupancy, and predictive maintenance.
24. **Integrated Wellness Studios** – Yoga, art, or mindfulness therapy spaces.
25. **Emergency Egress That Supports Calm** – Low-profile exits to reduce panic.
26. **Anti-Ligature Design** – Fixtures that minimize self-harm risk.
27. **Secure Medication and Supply Areas** – Controlled access to reduce diversion.
28. **Sustainable Materials and Clean Air Strategies** – Low-VOC and HEPA air filtration.
29. **Adaptive Lighting Design** – Tunable LEDs for circadian health.
30. **Mock-Up and Simulation Testing** – Early physical/virtual mock-ups to reveal inefficiencies.

31. **Zoned Thermal Comfort** – Orient HVAC zones for efficiency and satisfaction.
32. **Clear Infection Control Pathways** – Separate clean/soiled routes and strategic sinks.
33. **Shell Space for Expansion** – Rough-in unfinished areas for cost-effective growth.
34. **Mixed-Use Integration** – Locate near transit, housing, and social services.
35. **Interdisciplinary Team Reviews** – Include diverse stakeholders in charrettes.
36. **Embedded Digital Infrastructure** – Plan for telehealth and EMR integration.
37. **Continuous Design Feedback Loops** – Monthly user reviews for agile adaptation.
38. **Resident Artwork and Identity Expression** – Showcase patient-made murals/art.
39. **Warm, Durable Finishes** – Combine antimicrobial safety with tactile comfort.
40. **Healing Pathways** – Walking loops with wayfinding markers.
41. **Multi-Sensory Engagement Spaces** – Engage sight, sound, scent, and touch.
42. **High-Impact Entry Design** – Welcoming, trauma-informed entry experiences.
43. **Visibility Without Surveillance** – Maintain privacy while ensuring safety.
44. **Empowerment Through Wayfinding** – Intuitive layouts reduce anxiety.
45. **Connection to the Local Ecology** – Use native plants and materials.
46. **Continuous Outdoor-Indoor Transitions** – Covered patios and verandas as bridges.
47. **Discreet Security Integration** – Blend safety features into architecture.
48. **Dedicated Peer Support Services Spaces** – Peer recovery coaching rooms.

49. **Reduced Institutional Cues** – Eliminate harsh lighting and paging systems.
50. **Staff Sightline Mapping** – Ensure passive observation through planning.
51. **Discrete Service Entrances** – Separate delivery/waste routes.
52. **Non-Hierarchical Room Layouts** – Arrange furniture for equality in therapy rooms.
53. **Variable Seating Options** – Provide diverse, sensory-supportive seating.
54. **Staff Wellness Infrastructure** – Showers, daylight, and quiet rooms for staff.
55. **Participatory Design With Youth and Elders** – Tailor spaces via generational input.
56. **Generous Ceiling Heights** – Increase openness and reduce sensory stress.
57. **Decentralized Nurse Stations** – Smaller stations for rapport and faster care.
58. **Private Entry Zones** – Discreet arrivals for patients in crisis.
59. **Cross-Training in Design Intent** – Educate staff on therapeutic use of space.
60. **Facility Identity and Branding** – Build pride with strong visual identity.
61. **Lighting for Recovery Cycles** – Circadian rhythm-focused lighting systems.
62. **Art Therapy Integration** – Gallery walls and art therapy rooms.
63. **Mixed-Acuity Zoning** – Separate design for high- and low-acuity needs.
64. **Visitor Path Separation** – Clear, private routes for visitors.
65. **Decentralized Restrooms** – Frequent, single-use restrooms for dignity.
66. **Personal Lockable Storage** – Patient lockers for autonomy.
67. **Material Resilience & Aesthetics** – Durable yet attractive finishes.
68. **Transparent Quiet Zones** – Sound-buffered but visually open spaces.
69. **Active Circulation Design** – Avoid dead ends with looped corridors.
70. **Embedded Telehealth Infrastructure** – Private pods for teletherapy.
71. **Cultural Symbolism in Design** – Express belonging through local motifs.
72. **Reduced Seclusion Reliance** – Provide de-escalation alternatives.

73. **Dynamic Color Theory Application** – Use evidence-based color psychology.
74. **Rainwater and Nature Elements** – Add calming natural soundscapes.
75. **Cross-Program Collaboration Spaces** – Shared zones for care coordination.
76. **Lighting Zones With Dimming Options** – Patient control over brightness.
77. **Local Hiring for Construction** – Build pride and community ties.
78. **Integrated Transportation Access** – Support ambulances, buses, and bicycles.
79. **Site Resilience Planning** – Design for wildfire, flood, and quake risks.
80. **Community Gardens or Horticultural Therapy** – Gardening programs reduce depression.
81. **Distributed Nature Vignettes** – Place biophilic features throughout.
82. **Reflective Surfaces for Orientation** – Use mirrors/glass to improve mobility.
83. **Water-Inspired Design Motifs** – Flowing patterns reduce anxiety.
84. **Behavioral Emergency Response Zones** – Discreet spaces for urgent care.
85. **Interactive Wall Murals or Message Boards** – Patient co-created environments.
86. **Controlled Aromatherapy Zones** – Diffusers with calming scents.
87. **Mobile Therapy Pods** – Modular, flexible therapy stations.
88. **Use of Storytelling in Wayfinding** – Narrative-based signage and flooring.
89. **Predictive Analytics in Design** – Anticipate high-use areas from EHR data.
90. **Color Zoning for Cognitive Orientation** – Color-coded areas for clarity.
91. **Seasonal Light Programming** – Adjust lighting to seasons for circadian health.
92. **Textural Layering in Materials** – Diverse tactile surfaces to regulate senses.

93. **Transitional Patient Housing Units** – Independent-living practice units.
94. **Staff Collaboration Hubs** – Open workspaces for team communication.
95. **Interactive Technology Integration** – VR, biofeedback, and digital therapy tools.
96. **Quiet HVAC and Mechanical Systems** – Reduce mechanical noise impacts.
97. **Patient-Controlled Privacy Features** – Adjustable windows, sound-masking, and dividers.
98. **Lighting That Encourages Movement** – Use light pools to guide therapeutic activity.
99. **Design with Cultural Humility** – Flexible, inclusive spaces for diverse practices.
100. **Design for Long-Term Stewardship** – Durable finishes, flexible systems, and sustainable maintenance.

DESIGN PRACTICES FOR SUCCESSFUL OUTCOMES

1. DESIGN DOCUMENTATION BEST PRACTICES FOR COMPLEX SYSTEMS

Design documentation is the core communication tool among architects, engineers, builders, regulators, and the owner. Incomplete or uncoordinated documentation often leads to delays, change orders, cost overruns, and life safety violations.

Objectives of Technical Documentation

- **Regulatory Compliance** – Demonstrate conformance with licensure, ADA, fire/life safety, FGI, and local codes.
- **Construction Clarity** – Eliminate ambiguity and reduce RFIs.
- **Scope Control** – Clearly define finishes, equipment, and details to prevent scope creep.
- **Clinical Alignment** – Translate operational intent into built reality.

Best Practices

- Develop a **Room Data Sheet Matrix** linking each space to finishes, MEP loads, ligature compliance, and FF&E.
- Produce **Narrative Justifications** aligning clinical models with physical layout.
- Maintain a **QA/QC Peer Review Process** at 30%, 60%, 90%, and 100% design.
- Apply **BIM-based clash detection** for system coordination.

Risk Mitigation

- Track code references in annotated code sheets.
- Assign document control leads for version management and approvals.
- Pre-coordinate **high-risk zones** (medication rooms, seclusion suites) during DD.

2. COORDINATION BETWEEN DISCIPLINES FOR CONSTRUCTABILITY

Breakdowns between mechanical, electrical, plumbing (MEP), structural, and architectural teams cause costly field conflicts.

High-Risk Interface Points

- **Ceiling Congestion** – Coordinate ligature-resistant fixtures with ductwork, sprinklers, and lighting.
- **Wall Penetrations** – Route nurse call, security, and fire alarm cabling through rated assemblies.
- **Structural Reinforcement** – Backing for grab bars, millwork, and heavy fixtures.

Best Practices

- Hold **weekly discipline coordination calls** during DD and CD.
- Mandate **BIM modeling** with clash resolution before permit submission.
- Maintain a **constructability sign-off log** managed by the Owner's Advisor.

Risk Mitigation

- Tie product specs to procurement availability to prevent substitutions.
- Centralize issue-tracking with written closeout of items.
- Conduct **mock-up reviews** with all disciplines present.

3. INFECTION CONTROL, SECURITY, LIGATURE RESISTANCE, AND ACCESSIBILITY

Behavioral health projects demand design responses that address both clinical safety and regulatory mandates.

Infection Control

- Antimicrobial surfaces and seamless flooring.
- Negative pressure isolation rooms.
- HVAC zoning per FGI and CDC standards.

Ligature Resistance

- Anti-ligature fixtures: toilets, shower heads, faucets, door hardware.
- Reinforced walls and tamper-resistant assemblies.

Security

- Zoned access control by acuity level.
- Duress alarms and staff alert systems.

- Controlled egress and observation corridors.

Accessibility

- Universal Design compliance.
- Inclusive wayfinding, restrooms, and waiting areas.

Best Practices & Risk Mitigation

- Perform **ICRA assessments** during DD.
- Validate ligature compliance with cut sheets.
- Include security consultants in 60%+ drawing reviews.
- Conduct access flow simulations for emergencies.

4. DESIGN FOR HEALING, TREATMENT, AND RECOVERY

Facilities must support emotional safety, trauma recovery, and staff wellness.

Healing Design Elements

- Daylight, views, and natural connections.
- Calming palettes and residential-style furnishings.
- Acoustic comfort and noise reduction.

Supportive Space Planning

- Personalized patient rooms.
- Flexible therapy spaces.
- Defined family zones and private reflection areas.

Best Practices & Risk Mitigation

- Use **trauma-informed design checklists**.
- Employ curved forms and soft finishes.

- Avoid over-standardization that neglects cultural needs.
- Include former patients or peer navigators in reviews.

5. MANAGING EVOLVING USER NEEDS WITHOUT COMPROMISING SCHEDULE

Behavioral health projects must balance adaptability with disciplined timelines.

Best Practices

- Apply **universal room templates**.
- Allow deferred finish/fixture selection when feasible.
- Use **soft openings** with systems simulation.

Risk Mitigation

- Lock in **schedule-critical decisions early**.
- Maintain **milestone-based calendars** tied to procurement.
- Align permit submissions with actual phasing.

6. OWNER REVIEW CYCLES AND DOCUMENT CONTROL PROTOCOLS

Strong owner participation ensures clarity, accountability, and decision-making discipline.

Best Practices

- Owner reviews at 30%, 60%, 90%, and 100% design.
- Include input from operations, clinical, safety, and finance stakeholders.
- Maintain a **decision log** with documented approvals.

Document Control Tools

- Cloud-based platforms: Procore, PlanGrid, Newforma.
- Role-based access with version control.
- Change logs with justification memos.

Risk Mitigation

- Assign a dedicated document control lead or Owner's Advisor.
- Track unresolved comments with risk rankings.
- Enforce structured RFI and submittal review deadlines.

CONCLUSION: FROM DOCUMENTATION TO DIGNITY - ELEVATING BEHAVIORAL HEALTH THROUGH DESIGN EXCELLENCE

THE STRATEGIC AND MORAL IMPERATIVE OF BEHAVIORAL HEALTH DESIGN

Behavioral health care design is not merely a technical milestone -it is a **moral and strategic responsibility** that affects lives, operations, and long-term system outcomes. Every wall, window, and walkway in a behavioral health facility carries the potential to **calm, protect, and inspire**.

Through thoughtful, **research-backed design**, abstract values like safety, dignity, and recovery are transformed into lived experiences.

WHY DESIGN MATTERS

When designed with intention, behavioral health facilities:

- **Foster healing** and emotional safety.

- **Elevate human dignity** through trauma-informed environments.
- **Serve as lasting community assets** that sustain value and adaptability.

EVIDENCE-BASED OUTCOMES

American Institute of Architects (AIA) Findings

- Trauma-informed, biophilic design → **30–50% improvement** in patient satisfaction.
- Flexible design strategies → **25% better adaptability** + **40% reduction** in renovation costs.
- Interdisciplinary stakeholder coordination → **2.5x more likely** to achieve operational goals.

Design-Build Institute of America (DBIA) Findings

- Early Owner's Advisor engagement → **43% higher on-time, on-budget delivery**.
- Integrated design teams → **50% fewer change orders** + **35% faster regulatory approvals**.
- Early-stage leadership & planning → **28% stronger lifecycle cost control** across behavioral health projects.

THE ROLE OF THE OWNER'S ADVISOR

The importance of a seasoned **Owner's Advisor** cannot be overstated:

- Improves team coordination effectiveness by **45%**.
- Reduces project risk exposure by **38%**.
- Ensures **scope clarity, budget discipline, stakeholder alignment, and regulatory readiness** from day one.

THE BIGGER PICTURE

This data tells a powerful story:

- **Design is not just compliance or aesthetics** -it is performance.
- **Design impacts safety and clinical outcomes** directly.
- **Design shapes human experience** -how patients heal, how staff work, and how communities engage with behavioral health care.

THE LASTING IMPACT OF DESIGN LEADERSHIP

Great behavioral health design begins with **leadership** -experienced architects, clinical planners, Owner's Advisors, and engineers who understand the stakes and align the built environment with therapeutic goals. These professionals guide each phase with **precision, empathy, and accountability**.

A facility that flows efficiently, adapts over time, calms the agitated, and elevates the overlooked -**that is the legacy of strong design coordination**.

DESIGN THAT PERFORMS

What distinguishes **high-performing behavioral health design**? It is:

- **Evidence-Based** → Drawing from research to inform both form and function.
- **Trauma-Informed** → Softening sensory environments to reduce agitation and restore agency.
- **Biophilic & Natural** → Harnessing daylight, fresh air, and green space to reduce cortisol and support circadian wellness.
- **Neurologically Attuned** → Supporting attention, rest, emotional regulation, and social interaction.
- **Operationally Sound** → Enhancing staff visibility, workflow, infection control, and safety.

- **Culturally & Clinically Responsive** → Reflecting community values and adapting to evolving treatment models.

MEASURABLE OUTCOMES

When these priorities converge, results are both **tangible and transformative**:

- **33% fewer patient safety incidents** (AIA Health Impact Report, 2021).
- **22% higher staff retention in the first year** (Center for Health Design Post-Occupancy Survey, 2022).
- **20% fewer behavioral escalations** in well-lit, calming units (Ulrich, 2020).
- **Increased stakeholder trust and community acceptance** (DBIA, 2023).
- **Greater operational readiness and reduced turnover** post-occupancy (AIA Facility Performance Insights, 2023).

A CALL TO DESIGN WITH PURPOSE

As we move from **Chapter 9 into construction and execution**, we must remember:

- **Design is the heartbeat of behavioral health infrastructure.**
- It shapes every experience within the facility -patients seeking stabilization, nurses balancing care and crisis, families searching for safety and hope.

Great design is more than a blueprint. **It is a blueprint for healing.**

Every window placed with intention, every corner made safer, every space that soothes instead of startles -these are not mere design choices, but **acts of systemic transformation** in mental health care.

In behavioral health real estate, **excellence in design is not a luxury; it is a necessity**.

Let us commit to designing not just buildings -but **better futures**.

Chapter 10

Entitlements, Permitting and **APPROVALS**

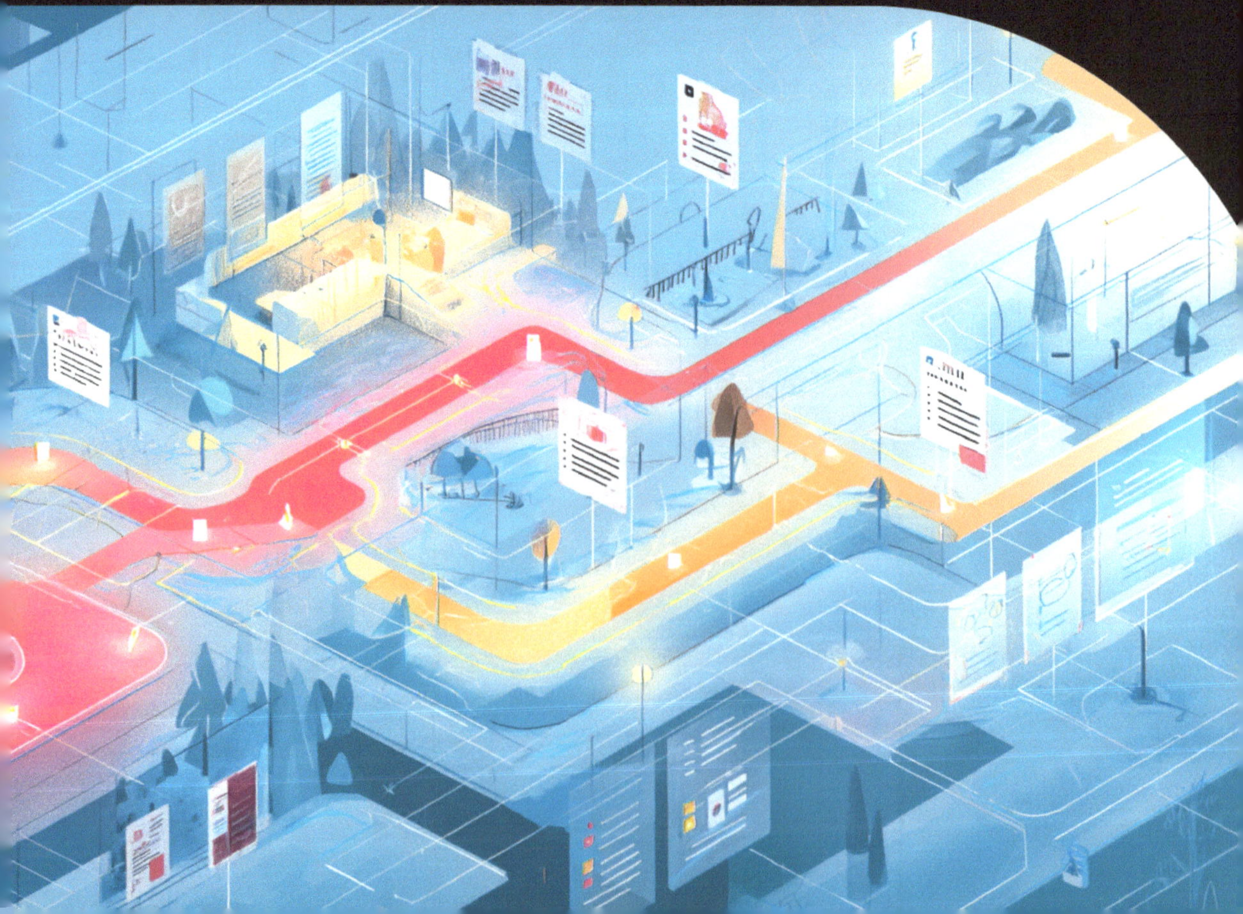

CHAPTER 10
ENTITLEMENTS, PERMITTING, AND APPROVALS

WHAT YOU WILL LEARN IN THIS CHAPTER:

- Navigating Jurisdictional Requirements and Politics
- State Health Department and HCAI Coordination
- Timeline Tracking and Fast-Track Permitting Strategies
- Environmental Assessments and Community Relations
- Proactive Engagement to Prevent Costly Delays

CHAPTER OVERVIEW

Entitlements, Permitting, and Approvals form the backbone of successful behavioral health facility development. This phase is where bold visions meet political realities, legal frameworks, and complex community dynamics. It is a space of both opportunity and risk, where strategic leadership, disciplined coordination, and communication mastery are paramount.

Great projects don't just navigate permitting; they master it. They do so with proactive engagement, integrated teamwork, and best-in-class project management. This chapter details how successful teams align with jurisdictions, anticipate regulatory requirements, minimize political resistance, and foster community trust. As Louis

Pasteur said, “Chance favors only the prepared mind.” In entitlements, preparation is everything.

Persistence turns regulatory friction into momentum. Treat every comment as a task that brings the goal closer. Behavioral health teams earn approvals by showing responsiveness and predictable follow-through.

Run a comment-to-closure system with weekly submittals and transparent updates to agencies and neighbors. Align CEQA, planning commission, and HCAI timelines. Show progress with side-by-side redlines so reviewers can say yes. If operating outside California, map this to your state authority and funding calendar.

FRONT LINE STORY #16. NAVIGATING POLITICS

> “Politics is the art of the possible.”
>
> OTTO VON BISMARCK

A project to build a new crisis residential facility was completely stalled. A key city council member, responding to intense NIMBY pressure from a small but loud group of constituents, was blocking our path at every turn. Public meetings were becoming hostile, and our timeline was in jeopardy. We knew a head-to-head fight would only harden the opposition.

So, we changed our strategy. We did our homework and learned that this council member’s signature issue was creating job opportunities for at-risk youth. We went back to our operational plan and, working with our future operator, built a robust local hiring and vocational training program directly into the facility’s model. We designed a partnership with a local trade school to offer internships in culinary services, landscaping, and administrative support, specifically targeting youth from the council member’s district.

We requested a private meeting, but instead of talking about zoning, we talked about partnership. We presented our “Community Workforce Initiative” and asked for his help in making it a success. The shift was palpable. He saw a tangible benefit for his community that he could champion, one that directly addressed his political priorities. He went from being our biggest obstacle to our most important advocate, personally guiding us through the rest of the approval process. We learned that navigating politics isn't always about winning an argument; it's about finding shared goals.

NAVIGATING JURISDICTIONAL REQUIREMENTS AND POLITICS

KNOW THE TERRAIN BEFORE YOU BUILD ON IT

Before drawing plans or launching announcements, a successful development team must **understand the local political, zoning, and regulatory landscape**.

Best Practice: Jurisdictional Mapping

Create a comprehensive matrix of:

- Zoning classifications and allowable uses
- Overlay districts and conditional use triggers
- Recent land-use disputes and council decisions
- Neighborhood associations and influential civic groups

Insight: Effective entitlement leaders build trust early by understanding stakeholder values, anticipating friction points, and communicating the project's **long-term social value**.

POLITICAL INTELLIGENCE AS PROJECT INSURANCE

Political risks are often invisible -until they become existential. Great real estate teams **neutralize these risks** by:

- Engaging city councilmembers and supervisors before applications are submitted

- Building relationships with planners, mayors, and community boards
- Tracking political cycles and elections that may shift land-use priorities

Project Leadership Tip: Assign a **Policy Liaison** to coordinate with legal counsel, Owner's Advisors, and public affairs teams to monitor political shifts.

STATE HEALTH DEPARTMENT AND HCAI COORDINATION

The Power of Early Engagement

Success with regulatory agencies begins before the first plan check. Permit-ready projects align **architecture, licensing, compliance, and health operations** from day one.

"Failing to plan is planning to fail." – Benjamin Franklin

Best Practices for Agency Coordination

- **Kick-Off Roundtable:** Host an all-agency meeting to set review timelines and clarify roles.
- **Working Groups:** Biweekly design + compliance syncs with legal, architects, engineers, and regulators.
- **Compliance Narrative:** Draft a master summary mapping all regulatory requirements to design features.

Integrating Project Management Tools

- Use Smartsheet, Asana, or similar to assign and track HCAI tasks.
- Maintain a **live HCAI checklist** with submission dates, next steps, and responsible parties.
- Owner's Advisor leads system management with design + legal support.

TIMELINE TRACKING & FAST-TRACK PERMITTING STRATEGIES

"You can't build a reputation on what you are going to do." – Henry Ford

Time is Money -and Credibility

Permitting delays cost more than capital: they erode trust, morale, and momentum.

Keys to Momentum:

- **Realistic Scheduling:** Build buffers, anticipate seasonal staff shortages.
- **Back-Scheduling:** Map deadlines in reverse from target construction start.
- **Permit Flow Charts:** Visualize dependencies between discretionary and ministerial permits.

Fast-Track Execution Strategies

- Select sites already zoned for healthcare/institutional use.
- Submit for multiple permits in parallel (e.g., CUP + OSHPD).
- Use pre-approved design templates.
- Build relationships with trusted third-party reviewers.

Team Practice: Hold **weekly permitting huddles** led by the Owner's Advisor to flag red risks, resolve bottlenecks, and prepare for agency interactions.

ENVIRONMENTAL ASSESSMENTS & COMMUNITY RELATIONS

Environmental Review as a Design Tool

Instead of treating environmental regulations as hurdles, leverage them to:

- Optimize site design

- Justify traffic calming and stormwater strategies
- Strengthen site resilience with consultant expertise

Best Practice: Integrate **CEQA/NEPA consultants** during conceptual design.

- Early Phase I & II ESAs prevent discovery-phase surprises.
- Proactive assessments reinforce community trust and long-term sustainability.

COMMUNITY ENGAGEMENT: LEADERSHIP IN ACTION

> "People don't care how much you know until they know how much you care."
>
> THEODORE ROOSEVELT

REAL ESTATE ENGAGEMENT FRAMEWORK

Successful community engagement builds trust, reduces opposition, and strengthens long-term project viability.

Key Steps:

- **Identify stakeholders early:** residents, businesses, schools, nonprofits
- **Develop a Community Relations Plan** with measurable outreach goals
- **Host listening sessions & open forums** to gather community feedback
- **Use visual communication tools** (3D renderings, flythroughs, diagrams) to explain benefits
- **Appoint a Community Liaison** to serve as the consistent point of contact

Case Example – San Mateo:

A project team created a **"Neighborhood Advisory Council"** to review design decisions and co-create a community art wall. As a result, **public opposition dropped by 60%** after their inclusion.

PROACTIVE ENGAGEMENT TO PREVENT COSTLY DELAYS

Where Projects Go Off Track

- Unclear internal roles and responsibilities
- Poorly managed communications with regulators
- Conflicts between architectural design and licensing regulations
- Inconsistent public narratives from team members

Strategic Coordination Systems

- Develop an **integrated action register** for all permit-related tasks
- Track **agency comments, decisions, and follow-ups** in real time
- Implement a **communications protocol** to ensure consistent messaging across architects, legal counsel, and community representatives

OWNER'S ADVISOR AS INTEGRATION LEADER

The Owner's Advisor plays a critical role in ensuring alignment across stakeholders and maintaining project momentum.

Responsibilities:

- Chairs **weekly entitlement coordination calls**
- Leads **milestone check-ins** against the master entitlement schedule
- Facilitates **early resolution** of design or regulatory conflicts
- Escalates unresolved risks to the Owner with recommended solutions

> "The strength of the team is each individual member. The strength of each member is the team."
>
> PHIL JACKSON

CONCLUSION: ENTITLEMENT AS STRATEGIC ADVANTAGE

The entitlement and permitting phase is not a hoop to jump through. It's an opportunity to build legitimacy, strengthen partnerships, and sharpen your project's focus. With excellent leadership, tight coordination, and stakeholder intelligence, it becomes a launchpad, not a landmine.

Real estate development is never a solo act. It's a symphony of disciplines, personalities, and pressures. The Owner's Advisor is the conductor, and success depends on their ability to keep everyone in harmony.

Closing Insight:

> "Risk comes from not knowing what you're doing."
>
> WARREN BUFFETT

In behavioral health development, what you don't know in entitlements can delay you for years. But what you do know, and prepare for, can accelerate delivery, reduce costs, and deliver facilities that heal, inspire, and last.

In the next chapter, we move from regulatory navigation to best practices of RE Development, where contracts are written, teams are assembled, and the stage is set for breaking ground.

PART THREE
ACCELERATION, TALENT, EXCELLENCE

Chapter 11

BEST PRACTICES for Rapid Delivery

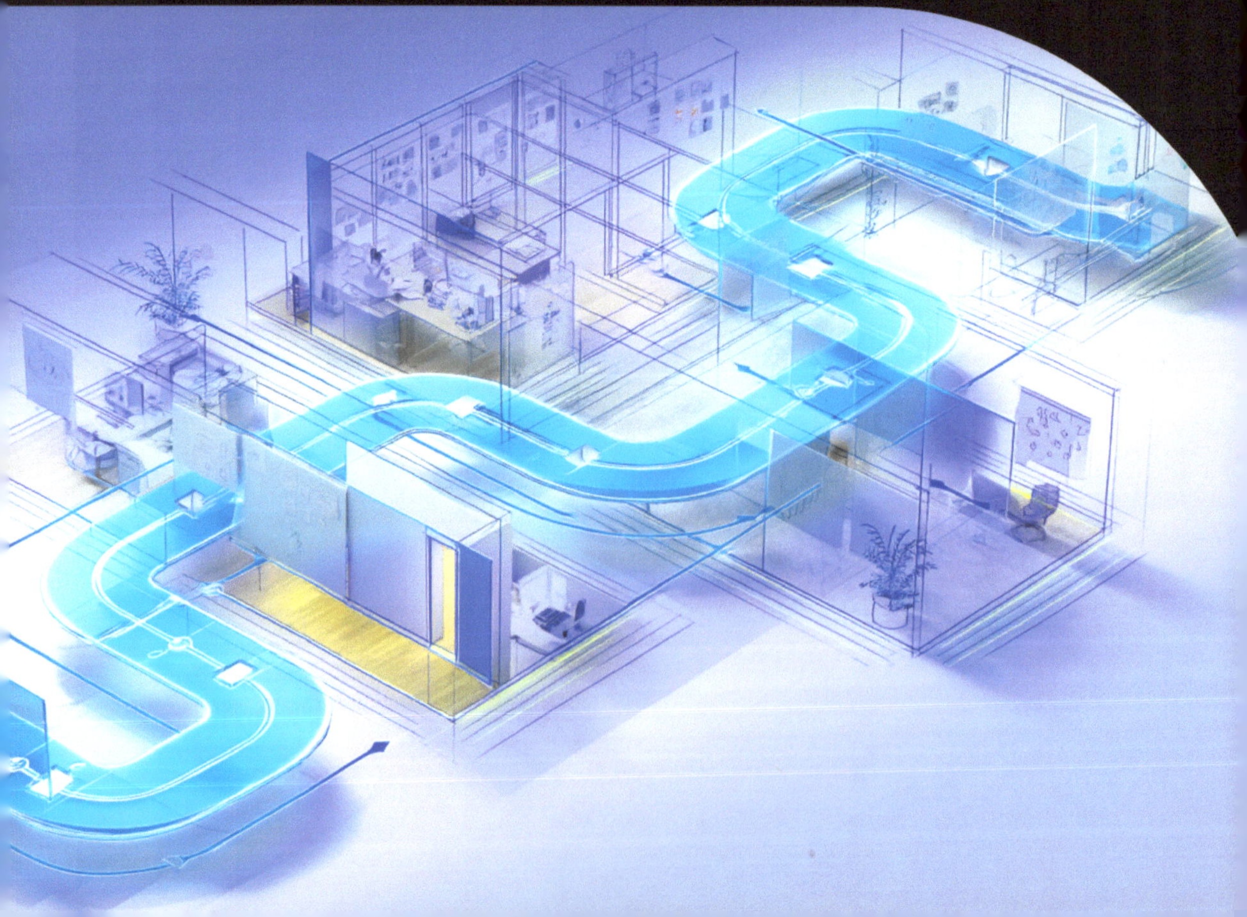

CHAPTER 11
BEST PRACTICES OF SUCCESSFUL BEHAVIORAL HEALTH REAL ESTATE DEVELOPMENT

WHAT YOU WILL LEARN IN THIS CHAPTER:

- Key Support, Teamwork, Vision, Mission, Values
- 100 Best Practices for Successful Behavioral Health Real Estate Development
- The Importance of Expert Teamwork

Organized planning and decisive action make rapid delivery possible without sacrificing safety or dignity. Design the work, limit work in progress, and remove blockers fast. In behavioral health projects, speed is earned by clear priorities and a cadence that keeps decisions moving.

Turn mindset into a working system. Map the critical path, set a two-week decision rhythm, and run parallel workstreams with clear entry and exit criteria. Use short daily huddles, weekly risk reviews, and a visible board for scope, schedule, and budget. Protect quality with defined checks at each handoff.

FRONT LINE STORY #17. ACCELERATING TIMELINES

> "The best way to get a project done faster is to start sooner."
>
> JIM HIGHSMITH

We were tasked with delivering a new crisis stabilization unit on an incredibly tight, 12-month timeline to meet a state grant deadline. The traditional design-bid-build process would have taken at least 18 months. To succeed, we had to rethink our entire approach. We opted for a progressive design-build model and immediately brought the general contractor on as a partner during the schematic design phase.

This early collaboration was a game changer. While the architect was finalizing the interior layouts, the contractor was already working with our civil engineer to begin site grading and foundation work under an early permit package. We pre-ordered long-lead items like the HVAC units and generator six months before they were needed on site. The teams held weekly integrated project meetings, solving constructability issues in real time rather than through a slow RFI process. It was a high-wire act of coordination, but by overlapping design, procurement, and construction, we were able to compress the schedule dramatically. We received our certificate of occupancy with two weeks to spare, securing the vital funding and, more importantly, opening a desperately needed facility months ahead of what was thought possible.

KEY TEAM MEMBERS, TEAMWORK, MISSION, VISION, AND VALUES

Developing a behavioral health rehabilitation facility requires more than bricks and mortar. It demands a **carefully orchestrated team**, a shared commitment to mission, and an unwavering dedication to patient-centered care.

This chapter outlines **best practices** for:

- Assembling the right team
- Fostering a culture of collaboration
- Aligning every decision with mission, vision, and values

When these principles are followed, organizations can **streamline execution, mitigate risks, and ensure the facility meets both clinical and operational needs** -while staying on **budget, scope, and schedule**.

BUILDING THE RIGHT TEAM

A successful behavioral health development project depends on the **expertise, coordination, and alignment** of its key professionals. Each member must bring specialized knowledge while working within a **strategic collaboration framework** that defines clear roles, maintains momentum, and mitigates risk.

1. Owner's Advisor – The Essential Guide

The **Owner's Advisor** is the linchpin of behavioral health facility development. Acting as the owner's trusted representative, they ensure alignment of objectives, budget, mission, and operational strategy.

Best Practices:

- **Behavioral Health Expertise:** Must know regulations, trauma-informed design, and care workflows.
- **Strategic Problem-Solving:** Anticipates entitlement, design, and construction challenges.
- **Leadership & Communication:** Serves as hub across architects, engineers, legal, funders, and contractors.

2. Real Estate Attorney – Navigating Complexity

Behavioral health projects require legal precision across zoning, licensure, healthcare statutes, and contracts.

Best Practices:

- **Healthcare Real Estate Expertise:** Knowledge of mental health care licensing and public funding.
- **Proactive Risk Management:** Anticipates entitlement and transactional hurdles.
- **Transaction Support:** Manages site control, lease/purchase negotiations, title clearance, and agreements.

3. Developer for Hire – Orchestrating Full-Cycle Delivery

A **Developer for Hire** drives execution across all phases, delivering turnkey results on behalf of the owner.

Best Practices:

- **Behavioral Health Track Record:** Demonstrated success in licensed, trauma-informed facilities.
- **Full-Scope Management:** Handles pre-development, permitting, financing, scheduling, and accounting.
- **Collaboration with Owner's Advisor:** Aligns strategy and execution to prevent scope gaps.
- **Transparent Reporting:** Provides milestone updates, cost forecasts, and contingency plans.
- **Operational Readiness:** Ensures facilities are license-, staff-, and activation-ready on day one.

4. Architect – Designing for Healing, Safety, and Performance

Architects shape the **healing environment** through design choices that support dignity, recovery, and safety.

Best Practices:

- **Behavioral Health Experience:** Anti-ligature, egress, sightlines, patient dignity, flexible layouts.
- **Clinical Collaboration:** Programming informed by therapists, physicians, nurses, and peer advocates.
- **Future-Proof Design:** Flexible infrastructure for evolving care models and licensing changes.

5. Civil Engineers – Laying a Safe, Sustainable Foundation

Civil engineers design the **site infrastructure** that ensures long-term safety, sustainability, and compliance.

Best Practices:

- **Healthcare Infrastructure Skills:** ADA, seismic zones, utilities, access, and drainage.
- **Sustainability Integration:** Green infrastructure, stormwater reuse, low-impact site planning.
- **Team Coordination:** Infrastructure supports constructability and long-term operations.

6. General Contractors – Executing with Precision

The GC ensures facilities are built to the highest behavioral health standards.

Best Practices:

- **Behavioral Health Construction Experience:** Secure materials, hardware, inspections, and infection control.
- **Cost Control Protocols:** Transparent billing, value engineering, and disciplined change order management.
- **Commitment to Safety:** OSHA excellence, HCAI Inspector of Record coordination, and compliance leadership.

THE INTEGRATED TEAM ADVANTAGE

When carefully selected, **aligned in values, and empowered by clear communication**, these professionals form the backbone of successful development. Together, they transform vision into **vital, healing infrastructure** that advances both **clinical outcomes** and **community well-being**. A high-performing development team operates as a cohesive unit, ensuring that every aspect of the project aligns with the facility's mission and patient care goals.

Best Practices for Team Collaboration:

Establish clear roles and responsibilities to avoid confusion and ensure accountability.

Foster open communication; regular project meetings should promote proactive problem-solving and cross-disciplinary collaboration.

Implement conflict resolution strategies; address disagreements constructively, keeping the project's mission and patient needs as the guiding priority.

> "Be quick, but don't hurry."
>
> JOHN WOODEN

FRONT LINE STORY #18. BALANCING SPEED AND QUALITY

During a rapid delivery project, the pressure to move fast can often lead to compromises in quality. We were facing this exact challenge while renovating an old medical building into a behavioral health clinic. The schedule was aggressive, and the construction team, in an effort to accelerate the work, began installing drywall before the city inspector had signed off on the in-wall plumbing and electrical work.

As the Owner's Advisor, my role was to protect the project's long-term integrity, not just its timeline. I immediately called a halt to the work in that section of the building. It was an unpopular decision that caused a one-week delay, but it was the right one. We walked the inspector through the site, got the necessary approvals, and then allowed the work to resume. I then facilitated a meeting with the entire project team to reset our priorities. We established a "quality-first" protocol, requiring formal sign-offs from both the inspector and our team before any systems were covered up. While we had to find other ways to make up for that lost week, we preserved the quality and compliance of the facility. The experience reinforced a critical lesson: speed is important, but quality is non-negotiable. A project delivered on time but built incorrectly is not a success; it's a future liability.

DEFINING THE MISSION, VISION, AND VALUES

1) ESTABLISH A CLEAR VISION

A behavioral health facility should hold a long term vision centered on patient care, community well being, and financial sustainability.

Best practices

- Align the vision with evidence based behavioral health models
- Engage clinicians, patients, and community members in visioning
- Translate vision into measurable goals for outcomes, operations, and finance

2) DRIVE THE MISSION FORWARD

The mission is the compass for every decision, from site selection to service delivery.

Best practices

- Communicate the mission to all team members and partners
- Embed the mission in layout, services, staffing, and daily operations
- Commit to community engagement to expand access and trust

3) UPHOLD CORE HUMAN VALUES

Facilities should embody dignity, respect, inclusivity, and patient empowerment.

Best practices

- Design for healing and comfort with warm, non institutional environments
- Prioritize cultural competency and language access
- Invest in staff training for trauma informed, compassionate care

CASE STUDIES IN BEHAVIORAL HEALTH DEVELOPMENT EXCELLENCE

CASE STUDY 1: LOS ANGELES COUNTY MENTAL HEALTH URGENT CARE CENTER

Challenge: The county lacked an efficient crisis intervention facility, leading to long wait times in emergency departments.

Solution: Developed a specialized urgent care center with calming interiors, crisis intervention rooms, and secure outdoor areas.

Outcome: 47% reduction in ER psychiatric holds within the first year of operation.

CASE STUDY 2: SAN FRANCISCO BEHAVIORAL HEALTH HEALING CENTER

Challenge: Outdated facilities produced poor patient experiences and limited service capacity.

Solution: Built a new center integrating biophilic design, trauma-informed principles, and flexible therapy spaces.

Outcome: Higher patient engagement and improved staff retention due to the enhanced healing environment.

CASE STUDY CONCLUSIONS

- World class behavioral health facilities require a strategic team, interdisciplinary collaboration, and mission driven outcomes.
- Best practices in team selection, teamwork, and value based decision making produce safe, effective, healing centered environments.
- With expert leadership, innovative design, and shared dedication to excellence, these facilities set new benchmarks for treatment and community impact.

"Problems are not stop signs, they are guidelines."

ROBERT H. SCHULLER

FRONT LINE STORY # 19. PROACTIVE PROBLEM SOLVING

During the due diligence for a site, we knew from experience that the local fire marshal was notoriously strict about emergency vehicle access for new healthcare facilities. The official process was to submit our plans and wait for a formal review, but that felt like a gamble. A rejection at that stage could set us back six months.

As the Owner's Advisor, I insisted on a proactive approach. We scheduled a pre-application meeting with the fire marshal, bringing our conceptual site plans and a list of specific questions. He was initially skeptical, but appreciated being consulted early. As he reviewed our plans, he pointed out a critical flaw in our proposed fire lane turning radius that, due to a recent code update we had missed, would have guaranteed a denial. He even sketched a solution on our plans, showing how we could reconfigure a retaining wall and adjust the parking layout to meet the new standard.

We walked out of that one-hour meeting with the key to unlocking our permit. Our engineering team made the changes, and when we formally submitted our application months later, it sailed through the fire department review without a single comment. That proactive meeting, which took only a few hours to prepare for, saved us from a costly six-month redesign and resubmittal cycle, keeping our grant-funded project on its tight schedule.

"Leadership is not about being in charge. It is about taking care of those in your charge."- Simon Sinek

TOP 100 BEST PRACTICES FOR SUCCESSFULLY DEVELOPING, PLANNING, DESIGNING, PERMITTING, CONSTRUCTING, AND MANAGING RISK IN BEHAVIORAL HEALTH REAL ESTATE IN CALIFORNIA

I. PRE-DEVELOPMENT AND STRATEGIC PLANNING

Site Selection and Feasibility Analysis (1–10)

1. **Conduct a Market Needs Assessment** – Analyze demographics, service gaps, and local demand.
2. **Evaluate Accessibility & Proximity to Services** – Choose sites near transit, hospitals, and emergency services.
3. **Confirm Zoning & Land Use Regulations** – Engage planning departments early to identify constraints.
4. **Secure Community & Stakeholder Support** – Build trust through early engagement with neighbors and officials.
5. **Analyze Infrastructure Readiness** – Assess utilities, roads, and environmental limitations.
6. **Mitigate Land Use & Permitting Risks** – Plan proactively for conflicts before purchase.
7. **Ensure Financial Feasibility** – Develop a pro forma with cost, revenue, and risk analysis.
8. **Plan for Scalability & Expansion** – Choose sites with room to grow.
9. **Assess Environmental & Geotechnical Conditions** – Conduct soil, seismic, and environmental studies.

10. **Appoint an Owner's Advisor Early** – Mitigate risks and guide approvals from day one.

Regulatory Approvals and Permitting (11–20)

1. **Map Local, State & Federal Compliance** – Identify all regulatory requirements upfront.
2. **Engage Local Officials Proactively** – Build relationships to accelerate approvals.
3. **Develop a Permitting Timeline** – Align permitting with construction milestones.
4. **Secure Conditional Use Permits (CUPs) Early** – Resolve zoning exceptions before design.
5. **Obtain OSHPD/HCAI Approvals** – Ensure compliance with healthcare facility standards.
6. **Prepare for CEQA/NEPA Reviews** – Anticipate delays and mitigate environmental risks.
7. **Streamline Building Permits & Inspections** – Use consultants to avoid bottlenecks.
8. **Align With Fire & Safety Codes** – Collaborate with fire marshals early.
9. **Plan for Accessibility Compliance (ADA & CBC)** – Design inclusively from the start.
10. **Leverage Expedited Permitting Programs** – Tap into incentives for behavioral health projects.

II. BEHAVIORAL HEALTH FACILITY DESIGN AND PLANNING

Patient-Centered and Trauma-Informed Design (21–30)

1. **Create a Welcoming, Non-Institutional Environment** – Design for dignity and comfort.
2. **Maximize Natural Light & Open Space** – Reduce stress with daylight and outdoor access.

3. **Use Calming Colors & Materials** – Support healing through warm tones.
4. **Incorporate Soundproofing & Noise Control** – Protect patients from auditory stress.
5. **Provide Private & Semi-Private Rooms** – Balance dignity and supervision.
6. **Design for Behavioral Health Safety** – Anti-ligature fixtures, impact-resistant surfaces.
7. **Include Outdoor Healing Spaces** – Gardens, walking loops, and green courtyards.
8. **Ensure Flexible Treatment Areas** – Adapt to evolving care models.
9. **Separate High- and Low-Acuity Zones** – Tailor environments to patient needs.
10. **Include Family & Visitor Areas** – Support recovery with family involvement.

Staff Efficiency & Security Design (31–40)

1. **Optimize Staff Workflow** – Reduce travel distances within layouts.
2. **Implement Secure, Non-Restrictive Access** – Balance safety and openness.
3. **Design Clear Sightlines** – Enable supervision while preserving privacy.
4. **Incorporate Safe Rooms & De-Escalation Areas** – Provide calming crisis spaces.
5. **Use Durable, Low-Maintenance Materials** – Lower lifecycle costs.
6. **Design Compliant Emergency Exits & Routes** – Clear, safe, and intuitive.
7. **Balance Security with a Healing Atmosphere** – Avoid punitive aesthetics.
8. **Integrate Smart Monitoring Technology** – Subtle, non-intrusive surveillance.
9. **Standardize Patient Room Layouts** – Improve efficiency and familiarity.
10. **Include Staff Wellness Areas** – Prioritize caregiver recovery and morale.

III. CONSTRUCTION & DEVELOPMENT BEST PRACTICES

Construction Planning & Execution (41–50)

1. **Select Experienced Behavioral Health Contractors** – Avoid costly learning curves.
2. **Use Modular & Prefabricated Solutions** – Speed up delivery and reduce disruption.
3. **Implement Strict Cost Controls** – Track budgets and change orders closely.
4. **Conduct Pre-Construction Regulatory Reviews** – Prevent compliance delays.
5. **Phase Construction for Minimal Disruption** – Especially in active healthcare campuses.
6. **Pre-Test Mechanical & Safety Systems** – Avoid licensing delays from failures.
7. **Monitor Supply Chain & Material Risks** – Secure critical items early.
8. **Conduct Regular Quality Inspections** – Maintain construction integrity.
9. **Plan for Commissioning & Post-Construction Tuning** – Ensure systems work as intended.
10. **Maintain Contingency Budgets** – Anticipate surprises and mitigate risk.

IV. OPERATIONS & FACILITY MANAGEMENT

Staffing & Workforce Planning (51–60)

1. **Develop Recruitment Pipelines** – Partner with schools and training programs.
2. **Train Staff in Trauma-Informed Care** – Embed best practices into patient care.
3. **Create Retention Strategies** – Offer competitive pay and wellness benefits.

4. **Ensure Adequate Staff Ratios** – Stay compliant and safe.
5. **Invest in Continuous Training** – Keep staff current with evolving standards.
6. **Provide Leadership Development** – Build strong facility managers.
7. **Develop Incident Reporting Systems** – Track, analyze, and resolve safety concerns.
8. **Ensure Multilingual & Culturally Competent Services** – Meet diverse patient needs.
9. **Foster Interdisciplinary Collaboration** – Encourage cross-team communication.
10. **Offer Employee Assistance Programs (EAPs)** – Support staff mental health.

V. LONG-TERM SUSTAINABILITY & COMMUNITY ENGAGEMENT

Community Partnerships & Advocacy (61–80)

1. **Engage Law Enforcement & First Responders** – Coordinate for crisis situations.
2. **Partner With Social Services** – Link patients to housing, jobs, and resources.
3. **Host Community Advisory Meetings** – Build transparency and trust.
4. **Educate the Public** – Reduce stigma with outreach campaigns.
5. **Develop a Workforce Pipeline** – Collaborate with universities and apprenticeships.
6. **Provide Competitive Salaries & Benefits** – Retain skilled behavioral health staff.
7. **Create Burnout Prevention Strategies** – Offer wellness programs and flexibility.
8. **Require Ongoing Professional Development** – Certifications and CEUs.

9. **Foster a Mission-Driven Culture** – Build inclusivity and shared purpose.
10. **Train All Staff in Trauma-Informed Care** – Embed trauma awareness into culture.
11. **Build Succession Plans** – Prepare future leaders through mentorship.
12. **Develop Financial Sustainability Plans** – Long-range budget forecasting.
13. **Maximize Medi-Cal & Medicare Reimbursements** – Ensure compliance in billing.
14. **Apply for State & Federal Grants** – Leverage SAMHSA, HUD, HHS funding.
15. **Negotiate Value-Based Insurance Contracts** – Tie payment to outcomes.
16. **Incorporate Green Building Incentives** – Offset costs with state programs.
17. **Create Revenue Diversification Strategies** – Add outpatient services or leasing.
18. **Leverage New Market Tax Credits (NMTCs)** – Finance in underserved areas.
19. **Conduct Regular Cost-Benefit Analyses** – Improve efficiency without cutting care.
20. **Monitor Policy & Reimbursement Shifts** – Stay agile with changing laws.

VI. OPERATIONAL EXCELLENCE & PATIENT-CENTERED CARE

Patient Care & Quality Improvement (81–90)

1. **Develop Integrated Care Models** – Blend behavioral health, medical, and SUD care.
2. **Use Data-Driven Quality Metrics** – Track and adjust outcomes continuously.

3. **Standardize Patient Intake Processes** – Improve efficiency and accuracy.
4. **Foster Continuous Improvement** – Regularly refine operations.
5. **Ensure Timely Access to Care** – Reduce wait times with telehealth and scheduling.
6. **Train Staff in Crisis Intervention** – Prepare for de-escalation and emergencies.
7. **Expand Peer Support Services** – Leverage lived experience in recovery.
8. **Engage Families in Care Plans** – Provide education and resources.
9. **Develop Strong Discharge & Aftercare Programs** – Prevent relapse and readmissions.
10. **Conduct Patient Satisfaction Surveys** – Use feedback to improve care quality.

VII. INNOVATION & FUTURE-PROOFING

Technology, Innovation & Future Planning (91–100)

1. **Adopt Behavioral Health-Specific EHRs** – Improve documentation and compliance.
2. **Implement Telehealth & Virtual Care** – Expand patient reach.
3. **Invest in Smart Building Systems** – Automate HVAC, lighting, and security.
4. **Leverage AI & Predictive Analytics** – Anticipate risks and improve outcomes.
5. **Develop Cybersecurity Strategies** – Protect sensitive health data.
6. **Design for Changing Demographics** – Adapt to shifting populations.
7. **Integrate Wearable & Remote Monitoring** – Track patient progress beyond walls.
8. **Prepare for Policy & Regulatory Changes** – Stay proactive, not reactive.
9. **Plan for Public Health Crisis Resilience** – Ensure continuity in emergencies.

10. **Commit to Environmental Sustainability** – Reduce carbon footprint and operating costs.

True success in behavioral health real estate development is never the result of chance; it is the result of deliberate decisions, a shared mission, and a team that understands the high stakes and human needs behind every square foot of space. The most successful facilities are built not only with technical precision but with moral clarity, clinical foresight, and strategic coordination.

These projects succeed when the development team operates as a cohesive, multidisciplinary unit, where every partner, from the Owner's Advisor to the environmental graphic designer, knows their role and honors the mission.

Summary of Best Practices:

Align Mission, Vision, and Values:

- Embed patient dignity into every phase of planning, design, and execution.
- Establish a shared vision across all team members, from finance and design to construction and operations.
- Reinforce values through project rituals, stakeholder engagement, and milestone celebrations.

Assemble the Right Subject Matter Experts:

- Choose professionals who bring behavioral health experience, not just technical capability.
- Prioritize real-world experience in regulatory approvals, trauma-informed design, infection control, and integrated care delivery.
- Empower experts to lead, not just serve, within their domain.

Define Roles, Accountability, and Communication Protocols:

- Clearly map decision-making responsibilities.

- Hold structured weekly coordination meetings with issue tracking and resolution paths.
- Use centralized, cloud-based platforms for real-time document control and versioning.

Promote Operational and Clinical Alignment:

- Engage frontline clinical and operations staff early and often.
- Validate space programs with simulations, mock-ups, and scenario walkthroughs.
- Invite peer recovery experts and lived-experience voices into the design process.

Foster Cross-Functional Collaboration:

- Use interdisciplinary design charrettes and planning workshops.
- Train the team in behavioral health safety protocols, cultural humility, and trauma-informed approaches.
- Build strong partnerships with regulators, licensing agencies, and local stakeholders.

Track Performance, Manage Risks, and Celebrate Wins:

- Monitor KPIs tied to schedule, budget, compliance, and readiness.
- Maintain risk registers with mitigation strategies and assigned owners.
- Acknowledge team contributions to foster morale and continuous improvement.
- Elevating Behavioral Health Through High-Performance Teaming

The behavioral health field is uniquely challenging. It demands a rare combination of empathy and precision, creativity and compliance, vision and execution. Buildings must meet exacting safety standards while simultaneously promoting warmth and healing. Development teams must integrate clinical protocols and construction logistics with equal fluency.

This duality is why expert teaming is so vital. Every phase of development, from site acquisition to facility activation, relies on intelligent collaboration between trusted professionals. And it is here that the Owner's Advisor plays a critical role: not as a passive observer, but as a dynamic leader of alignment, coordination, and accountability.

INTEGRATED THINKING, TACTICAL EXCELLENCE, AND LASTING LEGACY

Integrated Thinking in Action

Successful behavioral health projects are defined by **integration across disciplines**:

- **Architects** design with the operator's workflow in mind.
- **Contractors** build to meet clinical as well as structural goals.
- **Owners** do more than delegate -they steward the vision.
- **Staff, patients, and community members** contribute voices that are heard and valued.

When each role understands the others, the facility that emerges is not only functional but truly healing.

Strategic Vision Requires Tactical Excellence

Even the most inspiring mission will falter without disciplined execution. Tactical excellence means:

- Aligning **funding cycles** with **permitting deadlines**.
- Scheduling **clinical activation milestones** alongside **construction closeouts**.
- Balancing **innovation** with **licensability and cost control**.

Expert teams build this “muscle memory of excellence” through:

- Structured systems
- Early, decisive choices
- The discipline of documentation

Leadership, Learning, and Legacy

Behavioral health real estate is more than a business -it is a calling. To succeed requires:

- **Leadership that listens**
- **Processes that adapt**
- **Partnerships that endure**
- **Values that remain visible**, even amid construction chaos

Every project leaves a legacy. Some leave **scars** -built in haste, poorly aligned, quickly obsolete. But the best become **anchors of community healing, joy, and trust**.

These are the projects guided by mission-driven teams and advisors who understand what is truly at stake. As behavioral health needs rise and funding expands through state, federal, and philanthropic sources, the mandate is clear:

Now is the time to get it right.

Assemble expert teams. Align every task to mission. Coordinate with precision. Deliver not just a building, but a **sanctuary for recovery**.

“True healing begins the moment the environment supports it, and that begins long before the doors open.”

In the chapters ahead, we explore how these values are translated into operations, commissioning, activation, and community impact. But the foundation is here: in teamwork, expertise, and unwavering purpose.

Chapter 12

Rapid Delivery **METHODS** and Implementation

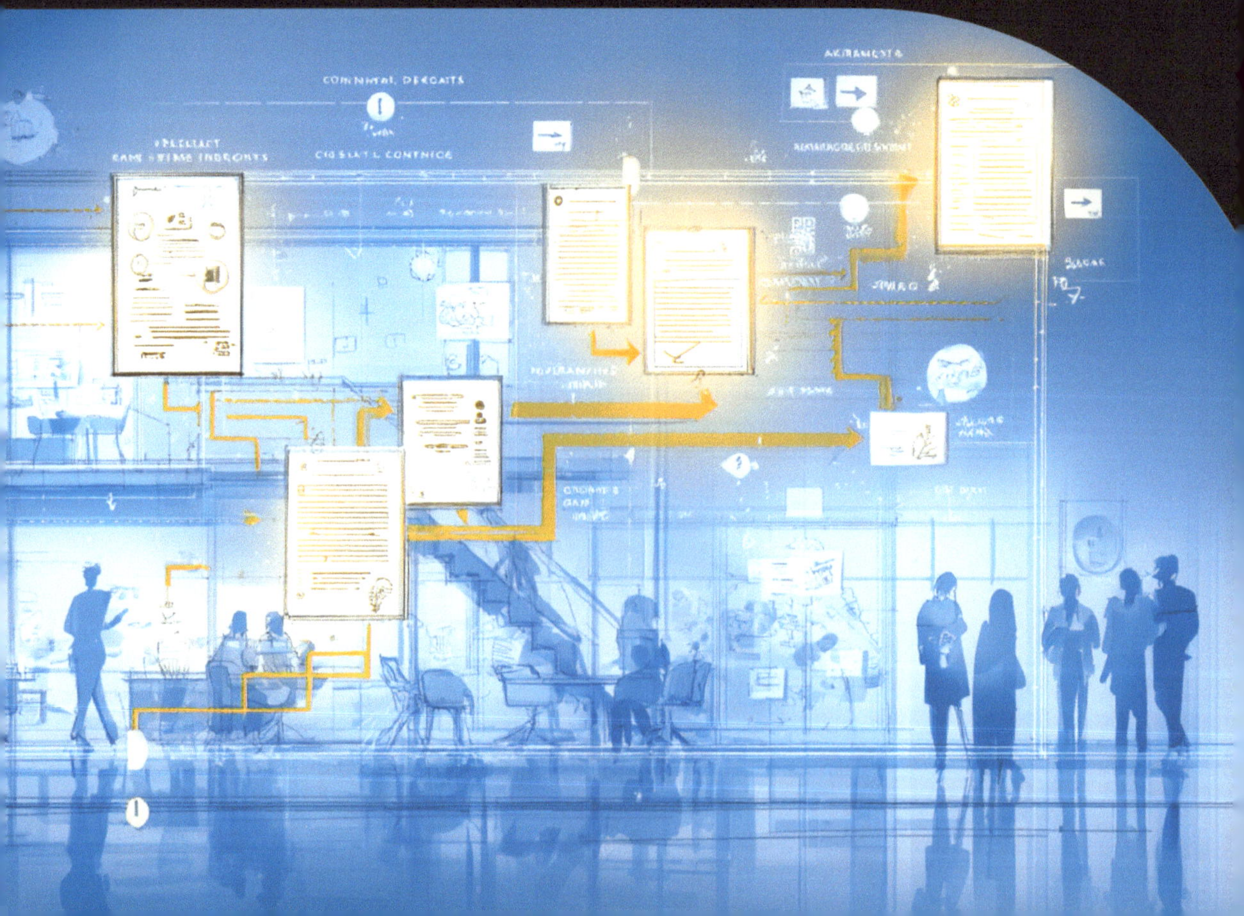

CHAPTER 12

ADVANCED STRATEGIES FOR ACCELERATING BEHAVIORAL HEALTH FACILITY DELIVERY WHILE MAINTAINING QUALITY AND COMPLIANCE STANDARDS

Initiative and leadership under pressure define the right delivery method and make it work. Choose a structure, name the risks, and build guardrails that keep the team moving when conditions change. In behavioral health, the best method is the one your team can execute with clarity and accountability.

Operationalize with a delivery method brief that spells out roles, incentives, and risk sharing. Set decision SLAs, co-locate when possible, and use target-value design to keep scope aligned with cost and schedule. Measure decision velocity and issue turnaround so you can see friction and remove it quickly. If operating outside California, map this to your state authority and funding calendar.

> "It's not that I'm so smart; it's just that I stay with problems longer."
>
> ALBERT EINSTEIN

FRONT LINE STORY #20. "FAST-TRACK SUCCESS"

We were awarded a significant state grant to build a new mental health urgent care center, but there was a catch: the funds had a strict 18-month expenditure deadline. A traditional development timeline would have taken 24 to 30 months, making the project seem impossible. Failure meant losing millions in funding for a community in crisis. The only path forward was a radical approach to permitting.

As the Owner's Advisor, I mapped out a parallel processing strategy. Instead of waiting for one approval to finish before starting the next, we initiated multiple processes at once. We submitted our application for a Conditional Use Permit (CUP) to the planning department while simultaneously beginning our environmental review under CEQA. At the same time, our architects, working with incomplete but well-defined schematic plans, held pre-submittal meetings with the building and fire departments. It was a high-stakes, coordinated effort that required constant communication between our legal team, consultants, and city staff. By fast-tracking the permitting on multiple fronts, we were able to get a shovel in the ground just six months after the grant was awarded. It was a testament to the power of proactive, integrated teamwork in the face of an impossible deadline.

RAPID DELIVERY BEST PRACTICES

The demand for behavioral health rehabilitation facilities is growing at an unprecedented rate, necessitating a faster, smarter, and more efficient approach to development. Delivering these facilities on budget, on scope, and on schedule requires a strategic fusion of innovative methodologies, cutting-edge construction techniques, and seamless stakeholder collaboration. This chapter outlines **20 proven methodologies for accelerating project delivery** while maintaining high standards of quality, safety, and functionality. These strategies are designed to help owners, developers, and healthcare leaders streamline processes, reduce costs, and bring essential behavioral health services to communities faster.

RAPID DELIVERY & STRATEGIC BEST PRACTICES FOR BEHAVIORAL HEALTH REAL ESTATE

1. Comprehensive Campus Master Planning

What It Is: Develop a master plan that organizes the layout, functionality, and integration of all facilities.

Why It Matters:

- Improves operational efficiency by reducing unnecessary travel.
- Enhances patient and staff experience through intuitive wayfinding.
- Facilitates phased construction for rapid activation of services.

2. Adaptive Reuse of Existing Structures

What It Is: Repurpose underutilized buildings (schools, warehouses, offices) into behavioral health facilities.

Why It Matters:

- Cuts costs by leveraging existing structures.
- Accelerates delivery by reducing permitting and foundational work.
- Promotes sustainability by minimizing demolition waste.
- **Case Study:** A decommissioned school in Ohio was transformed into a behavioral health campus in under 12 months.

3. Modular & Prefabricated Construction

What It Is: Use factory-built components assembled on-site.

Why It Matters:

- Cuts construction time by 30–50%.
- Reduces labor costs and weather risks.
- Ensures quality through factory precision.
- **Industry Insight:** Facilities have been delivered in half the traditional time using modular methods.

4. Flexible & Multi-Use Design

What It Is: Create versatile spaces that can adapt to evolving needs.

Why It Matters:

- Supports reconfiguration without major renovations.
- Keeps facilities "future-proof."
- Increases efficiency by serving multiple functions.

5. Fast-Track Project Delivery

What It Is: Overlap design, permitting, and construction instead of sequential phases.

Why It Matters:

- Speeds delivery by several months.
- Reduces bottlenecks with early approvals.

6. Integrated Project Delivery (IPD)

What It Is: Collaborative contract model that unites owners, designers, and builders from the start.

Why It Matters:

- Minimizes costly change orders.
- Improves communication and reduces errors.
- Encourages shared incentives for efficiency.
- **Data Insight:** IPD projects report 15–20% reductions in time and cost.

7. Sustainable & Resilient Design

What It Is: Use energy-efficient systems, eco-friendly materials, and sustainable methods.

Why It Matters:

- Cuts operational costs by 20–30%.
- Creates healthier environments.
- Enhances public perception and funding potential.

8. Proactive Community Engagement

What It Is: Involve residents, leaders, and advocates early.

Why It Matters:

- Reduces opposition and delays.
- Gains political and financial support.
- Encourages long-term community buy-in.

9. Zoning & Regulatory Readiness

What It Is: Work with local agencies to secure zoning approvals and compliance early.

Why It Matters:

- Prevents last-minute compliance issues.
- Avoids costly redesigns.
- Shortens approval timelines.
- **Pro Tip:** Consider preemptive zoning modifications for future expansions.

10. Phased Development Strategy

What It Is: Roll out high-need services first, then expand incrementally.

Why It Matters:

- Provides critical care faster.
- Allows staged financing and reduced risk.

- Adapts flexibly to demand shifts.

11. Efficient Site Utilization

What It Is: Maximize land with compact and multi-story layouts.

Why It Matters:

- Reduces land acquisition costs.
- Improves workflow and access.

12. Accessibility-Driven Design

What It Is: Incorporate ADA compliance and universal design from the outset.

Why It Matters:

- Enhances patient dignity and independence.
- Supports aging and diverse populations.

13. Rapid Prototyping & User Testing

What It Is: Use VR modeling and physical prototypes to test layouts.

Why It Matters:

- Reduces costly post-construction modifications.
- Ensures facilities are user-friendly for patients and staff.

14. Advanced Technology Integration

What It Is: Include EHR systems, telehealth rooms, and automation.

Why It Matters:

- Improves staff efficiency.
- Enhances patient experience.

- Reduces administrative burden.

15. Local Labor & Material Sourcing

What It Is: Prioritize regional contractors and suppliers.

Why It Matters:

- Supports the local economy.
- Cuts shipping costs and delays.

16. Emergency Preparedness

What It Is: Design for resilience against disasters, power outages, and threats.

Why It Matters:

- Ensures patient and staff safety during crises.

17. Continuous Quality Improvement (CQI)

What It Is: Use real-time data tracking during construction.

Why It Matters:

- Identifies inefficiencies early.
- Keeps projects on time and budget.

18. Scalable Design for Future Expansion

What It Is: Build spaces that can easily grow and adapt.

Why It Matters:

- Reduces renovation costs later.
- Supports evolving healthcare needs.

19. Stakeholder Communication Excellence

What It Is: Establish clear, transparent communication channels.

Why It Matters:

- Reduces disputes and misalignment.
- Improves accountability across teams.

20. Post-Construction Performance Evaluation

What It Is: Conduct structured post-occupancy assessments.

Why It Matters:

- Identifies lessons for future projects.
- Improves operations in real time.

PROGRESSIVE DESIGN-BUILD (PDB) FOR BEHAVIORAL HEALTH FACILITIES

The delivery of behavioral health facilities requires speed, precision, and compliance without sacrificing quality. **Progressive Design-Build (PDB)** offers a modern framework that emphasizes collaboration, flexibility, and phased delivery. When applied effectively, PDB accelerates timelines while ensuring facilities remain safe, therapeutic, and future-ready.

1. Early Stakeholder Engagement

What It Is: Involve clinicians, administrators, patients, and community members from the outset.

Why It Matters:

- Ensures the design reflects real-world operational needs.
- Builds trust, transparency, and community ownership.
- Reduces redesigns by aligning expectations early.

2. Integrated Project Team Formation

What It Is: Assemble a unified team of behavioral health architects, design-build contractors, and compliance consultants.

Why It Matters:

- Promotes seamless collaboration across disciplines.
- Reduces conflict between design intent and construction execution.
- Embeds safety and compliance expertise from day one.

3. Collaborative Design Process

What It Is: Use workshops, iterative reviews, and open communication channels.

Why It Matters:

- Surfaces challenges early and reduces costly late-stage changes.
- Encourages a culture of shared accountability.
- Improves efficiency through ongoing feedback loops.

4. Flexible & Adaptive Design

What It Is: Incorporate modular construction and multi-purpose spaces.

Why It Matters:

- Allows rapid reconfiguration for new treatment models.
- Supports both immediate needs and long-term adaptability.
- Reduces future renovation costs.

5. Regulatory Compliance & Standards

What It Is: Align with ADA, Joint Commission, state licensing, and anti-ligature requirements.

Why It Matters:

- Ensures safety, accessibility, and accreditation.
- Avoids costly delays tied to non-compliance.
- Builds credibility with regulators and funders.

6. Sustainable Design Practices

What It Is: Use energy-efficient systems, low-VOC materials, natural light, and outdoor healing spaces.

Why It Matters:

- Reduces long-term operational costs by 20–30%.
- Promotes healing and well-being through biophilic design.
- Enhances public perception and grant eligibility.

7. Technology Integration

What It Is: Plan for telehealth, EMRs, and smart building systems.

Why It Matters:

- Expands care beyond facility walls.
- Improves energy management and security monitoring.
- Future-proofs infrastructure for evolving technology.

8. Phased Construction Approach

What It Is: Deliver high-priority areas (e.g., emergency or inpatient units) first.

Why It Matters:

- Enables partial occupancy and early activation of services.
- Reduces downtime while construction continues.
- Provides flexibility in funding and staffing ramp-up.

9. Robust Project Management

What It Is: Set clear milestones, track budgets closely, and use proactive risk management.

Why It Matters:

- Prevents scope creep and cost overruns.
- Keeps teams accountable to schedule.
- Improves transparency with funders and stakeholders.

10. Post-Occupancy Evaluation

What It Is: Gather staff, patient, and stakeholder feedback after opening.

Why It Matters:

- Identifies opportunities for improvement.
- Measures performance against key metrics (safety, satisfaction, throughput).
- Informs best practices for future projects.

WHY PROGRESSIVE DESIGN-BUILD WORKS FOR BEHAVIORAL HEALTH

PDB accelerates delivery, reduces conflict, and strengthens outcomes by embedding collaboration, compliance, and sustainability at every stage. For behavioral health facilities, where time, safety, and adaptability are paramount, PDB is more than a project delivery method; it is a **strategic framework for building environments that heal, dignify, and endure**.

ADAPTIVE REUSE FOR BEHAVIORAL HEALTH FACILITIES

The rising demand for behavioral health services requires innovative, cost-effective, and sustainable real estate solutions. **Adaptive reuse:** the acquisition and rehabilitation of existing buildings offers a proven strategy to accelerate delivery, reduce costs, and mitigate risk while creating environments that promote healing and resilience.

ADVANTAGES OF ADAPTIVE REUSE

1. Accelerated Project Timelines

What It Is: Redevelop existing structures rather than building from scratch.

Why It Matters:

- Cuts months off project delivery.
- Leverages existing foundations, utilities, and infrastructure.
- Gets critical behavioral health services online faster.

2. Cost Efficiency

What It Is: Rehabilitate existing structures instead of ground-up construction.

Why It Matters:

- Reduces need for expensive sitework and foundations.
- Often eligible for financial incentives and tax credits.
- Provides substantial savings for limited healthcare budgets.

3. Sustainability

What It Is: Reuse instead of demolish-and-build.

Why It Matters:

- Minimizes construction waste.
- Reduces carbon footprint.
- Aligns projects with ESG (Environmental, Social, Governance) goals.

4. Customization & Flexibility

What It Is: Tailor existing buildings for behavioral health services.

Why It Matters:

- Creates therapeutic, culturally sensitive spaces.
- Allows adaptive design for specialized programs.
- Blends new health-focused features with existing community character.

BEST PRACTICES FOR ADAPTIVE REUSE

1. Comprehensive Site Assessment

- Evaluate structural integrity and environmental conditions.
- Confirm zoning and land-use compatibility.

2. Stakeholder Engagement

- Involve local leaders, neighbors, and advocates early.
- Consult with adaptive reuse and behavioral health design experts.

3. Behavioral Health-Specific Design

- Incorporate secure entries, passive observation areas, and anti-ligature fixtures.
- Maximize natural light, acoustics, and therapeutic layouts.

- Ensure compliance with ADA, Joint Commission, and HCAI/OSHPD standards.

4. Effective Project Management

- Use phased construction to prioritize urgent needs.
- Develop detailed cost models and track budgets closely.

5. Risk Mitigation

- Conduct structural, environmental, and legal due diligence.
- Secure proper insurance and contingency funds.
- Address issues like hazardous materials or seismic vulnerabilities early.

WHY ADAPTIVE REUSE WORKS

Adaptive reuse transforms underutilized schools, offices, or warehouses into **healing environments** faster and more affordably than new construction. By leveraging existing infrastructure, organizations can:

- Deliver services to patients sooner.
- Reduce costs and financial risk.
- Support sustainability goals while revitalizing communities.

CASE STUDY: TRANSFORMING A VACANT OFFICE INTO A BEHAVIORAL HEALTH CAMPUS

Background:

In 2021, a nonprofit behavioral health provider in Southern California faced urgent demand for inpatient and outpatient mental health services. Rather than pursue a multi-year new-build, the team identified a vacant 45,000-square-foot corporate office building located near transit, hospitals, and community resources.

Approach:

- **Comprehensive Site Assessment:** Engineers confirmed the building's structural integrity and seismic compliance. Zoning was adjusted with city support to permit healthcare use.
- **Adaptive Design:** Former cubicle spaces were converted into therapy rooms, patient lounges, and staff offices. Open atrium spaces became natural light–filled group therapy areas.
- **Safety & Compliance:** Anti-ligature fixtures, secure nurse stations, and clear sightlines were integrated without compromising a warm, non-institutional aesthetic.
- **Phased Delivery:** The ground floor crisis stabilization unit opened in under **10 months**, while the upper floors were renovated for outpatient and administrative functions.

Results:

- The facility opened **40% faster** than a comparable new-build project.
- Overall development costs were reduced by **28%**, largely by reusing existing infrastructure.
- The project diverted an estimated **1,200 tons of construction waste** from landfills.
- Most importantly, the center now provides care for **5,000 patients annually**, meeting a critical community need.

Key Lesson: Adaptive reuse not only accelerates delivery but also transforms overlooked buildings into **dignified, healing environments** that bring immediate impact to communities.

FRONT LINE STORY #21. INNOVATIVE DELIVERY MODELS

I vividly remember a project from early in my career that followed the traditional design-bid-build model. The plans were completed in a vacuum, sent out to bid, and the lowest-bidding contractor was hired. The result was a disaster. The contractor had no healthcare experience, the plans were full of constructability issues, and the project was plagued by costly change orders and delays. The relationship between the design team and the construction team was adversarial, and the owner was caught in the middle.

Years later, we embraced a progressive design-build model for a new facility. The difference was night and day. We brought the contractor and key subcontractors onto the team when the design was only 30% complete. They provided real-time feedback on cost and constructability, allowing us to make smart decisions early. When we encountered an unforeseen issue with underground utilities, the entire team, including the architect, engineers, and contractor, huddled together on-site and solved the problem in a single afternoon. There was no finger-pointing or lengthy RFI process. The project was delivered ahead of schedule and under budget, but more importantly, the collaborative spirit produced a higher-quality building. It proved that the delivery model isn't just a process; it's a philosophy that shapes the entire outcome.

IN SUMMARY: THE FUTURE OF RAPID BEHAVIORAL HEALTH FACILITY DEVELOPMENT

The rapid delivery of behavioral health facilities is not a theoretical ideal; it is a real, achievable objective grounded in the lived experience of today's best development teams. Yet, it is never easy. It requires navigating regulatory complexity, limited funding, tight labor markets, and an urgent public health crisis all at once.

Success comes only with an experienced, highly integrated team (a coalition of subject matter experts, builders, designers, and owners' advisors) who can move with speed, accuracy, and unrelenting focus. These professionals don't just execute a set of plans; they translate urgency into action. They balance code compliance with creative problem-solving and lead with a shared sense of purpose: getting critical care environments open, functional, and serving those who need them most.

Progressive design-build and adaptive reuse are not just delivery models; they are manifestations of a mindset -a mindset that says faster does not mean reckless and cheaper does not mean lesser. It means rethinking how we collaborate, how we plan, and how we execute. Looking ahead, the future of behavioral health facility development will be defined by our ability to embrace agile methodologies, tap into modular and digital construction innovations, and build deep-rooted partnerships with communities. Projects that once took years must now be delivered in months, and with the right systems and people in place, they can be. The truth is simple: rapid delivery is difficult, but it is possible. With the right team, the right tools, and a relentless commitment to outcomes, we can rise to meet this moment and transform underbuilt, underserved communities into hubs of healing, care, and resilience.

Chapter 13

Assembling the 25 Essential **PROFESSIONALS**

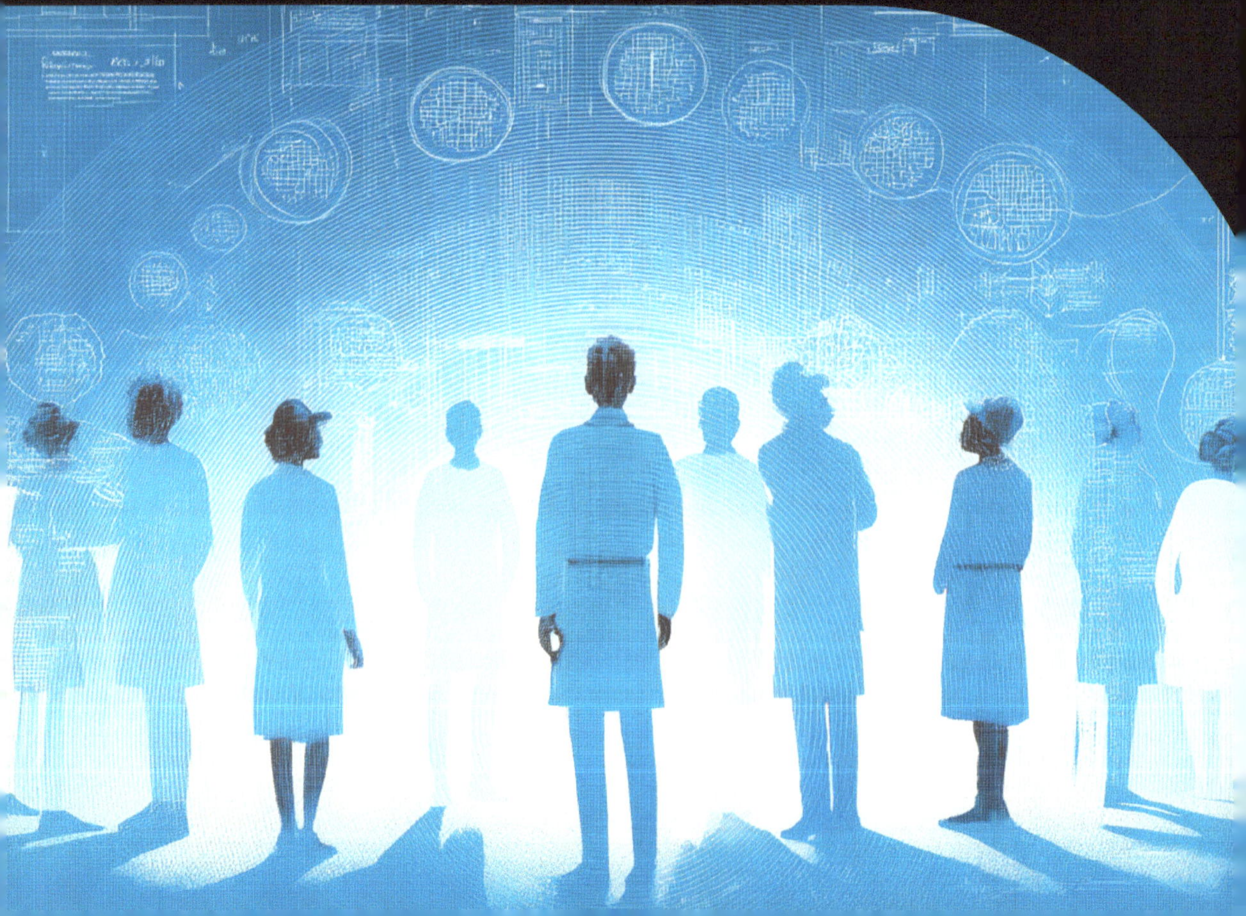

CHAPTER 13

"25 EXPERTS ON THE DEVELOPMENT TEAM: THE POWER OF EXPERTISE"

Mastermind and specialized knowledge make the 25 professionals a force, not a crowd. Assemble complementary expertise and give it a single aim. In behavioral health, the right voices at the right time accelerate permitting, improve design, and protect budget.

Build a visible roster and a cadence that turns expertise into outcomes. Define scopes crisply, set engagement windows, and run joint reviews for the hard intersections like safety, ligature resistance, and MEP coordination. Use checklists that prevent gaps and rework.

WHY SO MANY SUBJECT MATTER EXPERTS?

Developing a behavioral health facility is one of the most complex real estate endeavors, requiring precise coordination, strict regulatory compliance, and a deep understanding of patient-centered care. Unlike traditional commercial or residential projects, behavioral health facilities must seamlessly integrate healthcare regulations, safety considerations, therapeutic design principles, and operational efficiency. This level of complexity demands a highly specialized team. Each professional plays a critical role in reducing risk, maintaining compliance, and ensuring long-term operational success. Every subject matter expert (SME) contributes essential knowledge and skills that prevent costly mistakes, delays, or suboptimal facility performance.

At the center of this collaboration is the Owner's Advisor, the single most important expert responsible for aligning the team, ensuring smooth communication, and keeping the project within scope, budget, and schedule. The Owner's Advisor is not just a project manager but a strategic leader who integrates the expertise of all 25 professionals into a cohesive, well-executed development plan.

THE OWNER'S ADVISOR: THE KEY TO PROJECT SUCCESS

The Owner's Advisor is the owner's trusted subject matter expert and project steward, guiding every aspect of development from concept to completion. Unlike a general contractor or a real estate broker, the Owner's Advisor bridges the gap between the owner's vision and the technical execution by ensuring that all SMEs are working toward the same goals.

WHY THE OWNER'S ADVISOR IS CRITICAL

- **Expert oversight:** Ensures each subject matter expert contributes effectively, preventing misalignment and redundancy.
- **Risk management:** Anticipates and resolves issues early to reduce delays and change orders.
- **Regulatory compliance:** Monitors adherence to behavioral health regulations to avoid legal and licensing problems.
- **Cost and schedule control:** Keeps budgets tight and timelines realistic to protect financial and operational viability.
- **Stakeholder coordination:** Serves as the key liaison among the owner, agencies, designers, engineers, and contractors.

Without an Owner's Advisor, projects risk falling into cost overruns, schedule delays, compliance violations, and functional inefficiencies. This role is the linchpin that holds all other SMEs accountable and ensures a seamless development process.

THE 25 ESSENTIAL PROFESSIONALS FOR BEHAVIORAL HEALTH DEVELOPMENT

Developing a behavioral health facility requires expertise that spans vision, technical execution, compliance, operations, and community engagement. Below, the 25 essential professionals are organized into **five key categories**.

I. CORE LEADERSHIP & STRATEGIC OVERSIGHT

1. Project Owner / Developer – Defines vision, secures funding, and makes final decisions.
Why They Matter: The project's viability and direction depend on this role.

2. Owner's Advisor – Acts as the owner's right hand, aligning the team and monitoring budget, schedule, and compliance.
Why They Matter: Provides cohesion and accountability, preventing overruns.

3. Legal Counsel – Drafts contracts, manages risk, and ensures regulatory compliance.
Why They Matter: Prevents lawsuits, permit denials, and financial exposure.

4. Financial Manager – Manages budgets, funding, and forecasting.
Why They Matter: Financial stability is critical to project success.

5. Asset Manager – Oversees long-term property performance and operational efficiency.
Why They Matter: Ensures the facility remains financially sustainable post-construction.

II. TECHNICAL & DESIGN EXPERTS

1. Commercial Architect – Designs safe, functional, and healing facilities.
Why They Matter: Poor design creates inefficiencies and compliance risks.

2. Civil Engineer – Manages grading, drainage, and site infrastructure.
Why They Matter: Prevents flooding, instability, and zoning issues.

3. Structural Engineer – Ensures building safety and seismic stability.
Why They Matter: Protects patients and staff from catastrophic risks.

4. MEP Engineers (Mechanical, Electrical, Plumbing) – Design core building systems for efficiency and safety.
Why They Matter: Faulty systems cause outages and health hazards.

5. Lighting Specialist – Designs therapeutic and safe lighting environments.
Why They Matter: Lighting directly impacts mental health and recovery.

6. Interior Designer – Selects materials, colors, and furnishings for durability and calmness.
Why They Matter: Interiors affect stress levels and therapeutic outcomes.

7. Landscape Architect – Creates gardens and outdoor therapy spaces.
Why They Matter: Nature enhances recovery and offers safe healing areas.

8. Urban Planner – Ensures zoning and land-use compatibility.
Why They Matter: Prevents costly land-use conflicts.

III. COMPLIANCE, SAFETY & RISK MANAGEMENT

1. Healthcare Consultant – Advises on service delivery and operational standards.
Why They Matter: Aligns the facility with best practices in healthcare delivery.
2. Trauma-Informed Care Specialist – Ensures spaces support emotional safety and healing.
Why They Matter: Prevents re-traumatization and enhances patient dignity.
3. Regulatory Compliance Manager – Oversees adherence to healthcare codes and regulations.
Why They Matter: Avoids fines, penalties, and licensing delays.
4. Expeditor – Navigates permitting and bureaucratic approvals.
Why They Matter: Accelerates approvals, saving months of delays.
5. Operations Specialist – Designs workflows and daily operations.
Why They Matter: Prevents staff burnout and ensures efficient patient care.
6. Technology Specialist – Integrates telehealth, security, and EHR systems.
Why They Matter: Modern systems expand access and improve efficiency.
7. Utility Consultant – Secures reliable utility connections.
Why They Matter: Utility failures directly jeopardize patient care.

IV. FINANCE, MARKETING & OCCUPANCY

1. Marketing Specialist – Promotes the facility and builds awareness.
Why They Matter: Without visibility, the facility may struggle to attract patients.

2. Sales Representative – Develops referral pipelines and partnerships.
Why They Matter: Occupancy drives financial sustainability.

3. Real Estate Broker – Identifies and secures the property.
Why They Matter: Location directly impacts patient volume and accessibility.

4. Research Analyst – Provides market and demographic insights.

Why They Matter: Aligns services with real community needs.

V. COMMUNITY & STAKEHOLDER ENGAGEMENT

1. Community Relations Coordinator – Builds relationships with residents, leaders, and advocacy groups.
Why They Matter: Community buy-in smooths approvals and ensures long-term support.

THE POWER OF TEAMWORK IN REAL ESTATE DEVELOPMENT

Real estate development is a **multidisciplinary endeavor** that demands seamless coordination. The successful delivery of behavioral health facilities -on budget, on scope, and on schedule -depends on the ability of **25 top professionals** to function as a cohesive, high-performing team.

Teamwork as the Foundation of Excellence

Excellence arises when diverse professionals collaborate seamlessly. The **Owner's Advisor** plays a pivotal role in maintaining alignment across all experts, ensuring that each decision supports the project's mission.

Aligning Mission, Vision, and Values

A unified vision is the cornerstone of success. When all professionals share a common mission, the project benefits from:

- Greater cohesion
- Improved efficiency
- Purpose-driven execution

Comprehensive Scope Definition Through Collaboration

Defining scope requires early collaboration among **architects, engineers, compliance managers, and financial managers**. This approach:

- Prevents costly redesigns
- Reduces delays
- Ensures that operational needs align with financial realities

Interdisciplinary Schedule Management

Projects involve complex interdependencies. A collaborative scheduling process - guided by **expediters and construction managers** -helps the team:

- Anticipate bottlenecks
- Mitigate risks proactively
- Keep timelines realistic and achievable

Budgeting and Financial Oversight as a Team Effort

Financial health is not the responsibility of one person but of the **entire team**. When **financial managers, brokers, and contractors** work together, the results are:

- Reduced cost overruns
- Smarter allocation of resources
- Stronger financial accountability

Quality Assurance Through Team Commitment

High-quality design and construction are non-negotiable. A culture of excellence across all disciplines -from **interior design to structural engineering** -ensures the facility is:

- Safe

- Effective
- Durable

Engaging Stakeholders as a Unified Team

Behavioral health projects require buy-in from communities, agencies, and investors. A unified approach -led by **community relations specialists and legal counsel** -helps the team:

- Prevent opposition
- Build public trust
- Achieve seamless integration

Risk Management as a Collective Responsibility

Real estate development carries inherent risks. By collaborating, **compliance managers, urban planners, and technology specialists** create a resilient project that:

- Anticipates challenges
- Adapts to unforeseen events
- Protects long-term outcomes

A Team Mindset of Continuous Learning

The real estate landscape evolves constantly. Teams that embrace continuous learning through **knowledge-sharing and feedback loops** remain:

- Adaptive
- Innovative
- Competitive

Celebrating Success and Acknowledging Contributions

Every project is the sum of countless individual efforts. Recognizing achievements:

- Boosts morale
- Reinforces cohesion
- Strengthens long-term collaboration

> "Coming together is a beginning, staying together is progress, and working together is success."
>
> HENRY FORD

FRONT LINE STORY #22. "SYNERGY IN ACTION"

We were designing a therapeutic garden for a children's behavioral health facility on a tight, oddly shaped urban lot. The challenges seemed insurmountable. The architect was struggling to fit all the programmatic requirements into the space, the civil engineer was concerned about drainage on the sloped site, and the clinical director was adamant that the space feel open and safe, not cramped or enclosed.

The breakthrough came during a site walk with the entire team. As we stood there, the landscape architect pointed out a section of an old, non-structural brick wall at the back of the property. She suggested turning it into a vertical garden and a water feature. The civil engineer realized he could use the water feature to create a natural, gravity fed drainage system for the entire site. The architect saw how this vertical element could anchor the design, creating distinct "zones" for quiet reflection and active play without needing to build new walls. The clinician loved the idea of the calming sound of water and the therapeutic activity of gardening. In that moment, four different disciplines, each looking at the same problem from a different angle, created a single, elegant solution that none of them could have conceived of alone. That is the power of synergy.

> "The secret of success is not to do your own work, but to recognize the right man to do it."
>
> ANDREW CARNEGIE

BEST PRACTICES FOR TEAM FORMATION AND SUCCESS

Behavioral health real estate development requires **precision in team formation**. Every professional decision has downstream impacts on patient dignity, care delivery, and long-term sustainability. The right team is not assembled by chance -it is built through deliberate strategy.

Strategic Selection

- Vet candidates not only for their credentials but for their **behavioral health-specific experience**.
- Ensure each professional has a proven portfolio of relevant projects.

Hire for Chemistry

- Technical skills alone are not enough.
- Seek **team cohesion, shared values, and compatible communication styles**.
- A high-functioning team is built on both competence and chemistry.

Integrate the Owner's Advisor

- The **Owner's Advisor** acts as the strategic glue.
- Aligns all professionals to the project's mission.
- Anticipates and mitigates risks before they become costly.

Create Clear Roles & Accountability

- Define **who leads what** from the outset.
- Establish decision-making protocols.
- Clarify what success looks like at each project phase.

Embed Clinical Insight Early

- Include **clinicians, peer advocates, and operational leaders** in programming and design.
- Ensures facilities reflect real-world care delivery needs.

Foster a High-Trust Culture

- Projects run at the speed of trust.
- Establish communication norms and **resolve conflicts early**.
- Encourage transparency and accountability.

Align the Team to Mission & Impact

- Go beyond deadlines and budgets.
- Anchor the team in the **"why"**: addressing the urgent mental health crisis and delivering spaces that restore dignity and healing.

THE COLLECTIVE POWER OF EXPERT TEAMS

The best projects are never the product of **individual brilliance**. They are the outcome of:

- **Collective intelligence**
- **Cross-functional excellence**
- **Purpose-driven leadership**

Team selection is not just HR -it is **mission alignment**.

SUMMARY: PRECISION-SELECTED EXPERTS, INTEGRATED EXECUTION

In behavioral health development, the difference between a project that **merely opens** and one that **transforms lives** lies in the strength of its people.

- The **25 core professionals** are not just role-fillers; they are **mission-critical assets**.
- When strategically chosen, clearly coordinated, and empowered to work in harmony, they form a **development ecosystem** that delivers facilities which are:
    - **Compliant**
    - **Compassionate**
    - **High-performing**
    - **Sustainable**

Behavioral health projects demand **specialized subject matter experts**, not generalists. These professionals bring the insight, judgment, and commitment necessary to create healing-centered infrastructure that endures.

FRONT LINE STORY #23. FINDING THE RIGHT PARTNER

On a particularly complex renovation project, our original structural engineer was causing significant delays. They were unresponsive, and their designs were overly conservative and expensive. The project was at risk of falling behind schedule and going over budget. We knew we had to make a change, but finding the right partner midstream was a challenge.

Instead of just looking for a firm with a good resume, we looked for a partner with a reputation for collaboration and creative problem-solving. We found a smaller, local engineering firm whose principal was known for being a hands-on, solutions-oriented leader. During the interview, we didn't just talk about their qualifications; we walked them through our biggest challenges. Their team immediately started whiteboarding solutions right there in the room. We hired them on the spot. They integrated seamlessly with our architect and contractor, and within two weeks, they had value-engineered the design, saving us nearly $500,000 and getting the project back on track. It was a powerful lesson that the "right" partner isn't always the biggest or most famous firm; it's the one that shares your commitment to the mission and knows how to work as part of a team.

FINAL THOUGHT: PROJECTS END, BUT IMPACT ENDURES

The ribbon-cutting is not the end. It's the beginning of a facility's decades-long legacy. And that legacy begins with the people who planned it, designed it, and built it. When 25 expert professionals operate as one team with clarity, discipline, and heart, they do more than build buildings. They build hope. They build dignity. They build access to healing.

Let this be the standard going forward: Assemble not the largest team, but the right team. Equip them with trust, align them with a mission, and deliver not just real estate, but real care.

Professional **EXCELLENCE** in Daily Practice

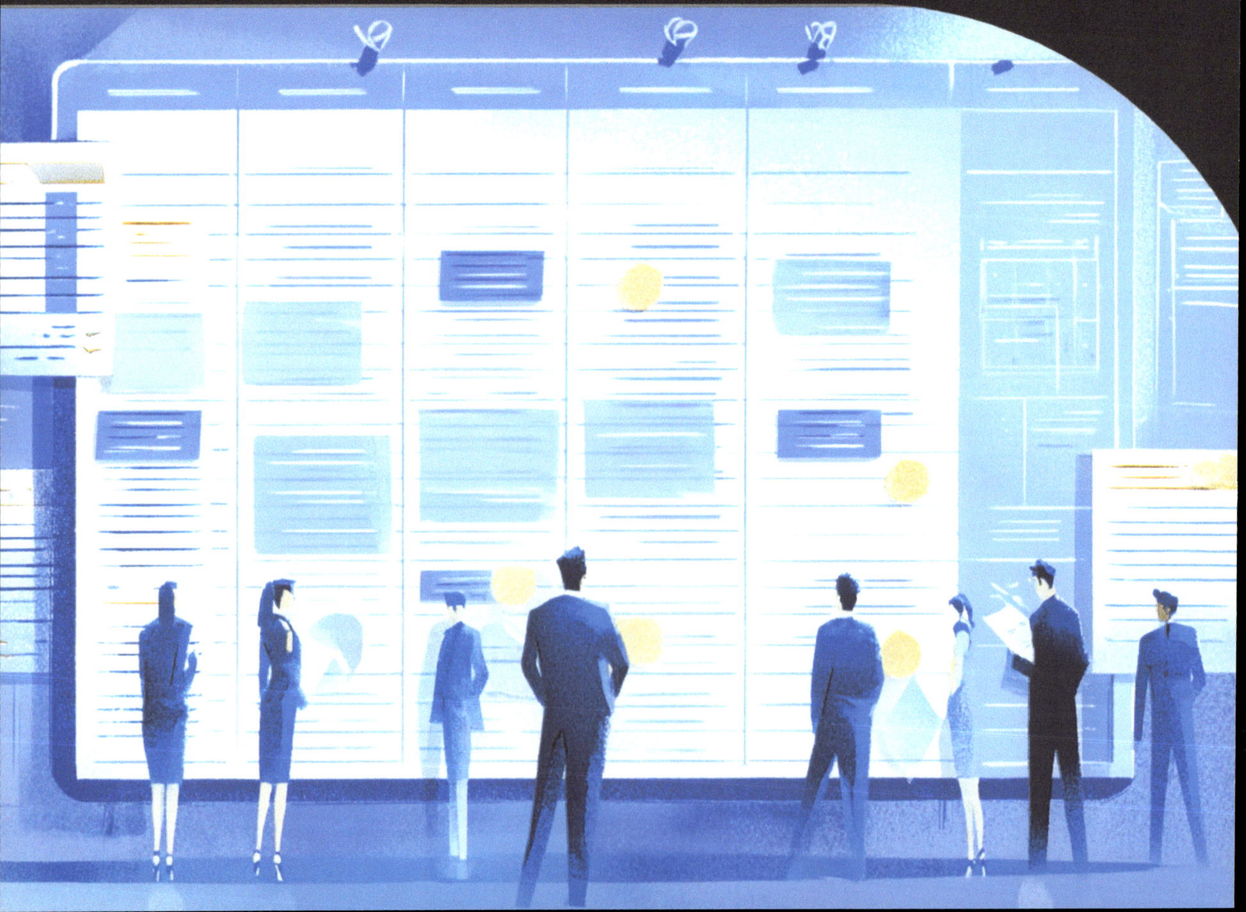

CHAPTER 14
PROFESSIONAL EXCELLENCE IN BEHAVIORAL HEALTH REAL ESTATE DEVELOPMENT

WHAT YOU WILL LEARN:

- Defining Standards of Quality
- The Power of Teamwork
- Stakeholder Support
- Owner's Advisors: Trusted Guides

Self-discipline is the habit that converts standards into daily outcomes. Keep promises to yourself and your team. In behavioral health projects, excellence looks like clean documents, on-time submittals, and field follow-through when stress is highest.

Turn mindset into rituals and tools. Start days with a 15-minute calibration, end with a five-minute clean down, and protect two 90-minute focus blocks per lead. Track the three most important for each lead and close loops daily. Make excellence visible so it is contagious.

Developing behavioral health facilities is a profound responsibility that requires unwavering dedication to quality, collaboration, and specialized expertise. These facilities are more than structures; they are sanctuaries of healing designed to support mental health and well-being. Achieving professional excellence in this field involves setting rigorous standards, fostering interdisciplinary teamwork, securing stakeholder support, and recognizing the indispensable role of experienced Owners' Advisors. These elements collectively ensure that behavioral health facilities operate at the pinnacle of efficiency and compassion.

PROFESSIONAL EXCELLENCE: DEFINED AND MAINTAINED

The foundation of professional excellence is an unwavering dedication to quality, rigorously defined and consistently upheld throughout all phases of development.

"Specialized subject matter expertise"

The development of behavioral health facilities necessitates the synergy of diverse expertise. Successful projects integrate insights from real estate developers, mental health professionals, healthcare architects, clinical operations specialists, and community planners. This multidisciplinary approach ensures that facilities are not only structurally sound but also conducive to optimal therapeutic outcomes.

> "Quality is not an act, it is a habit."
>
> ARISTOTLE

FRONT LINE STORY #24. DEFINING QUALITY

During the design phase of an adolescent psychiatric facility, we were specifying the door hardware for patient rooms. The budget was tight, and the team was considering a standard, institutional-grade, anti-ligature hardware set that, while compliant, was cold, metallic, and sterile. It met the technical definition of quality by being safe and durable, but it failed to meet the human definition of quality.

I remember our lead clinician pausing the meeting and asking, "Is this a space where we would want our own child to heal?" That question shifted the entire conversation. We spent the next week researching alternatives and found a newer product line from a European manufacturer. It was more expensive, but it was designed with warm, wood-like finishes and a softer, more residential feel while still meeting the highest safety and ligature-resistance standards. We presented a cost-benefit analysis to the owner, framing the additional expense not as a cost but as an investment in patient dignity. They approved it immediately. A year after the facility opened, the clinical director told me that the simple act of having a warm, non-institutional door handle made a noticeable difference in reducing patient anxiety upon entering their rooms. That is the definition of quality: when every detail, no matter how small, serves the mission of healing.

"EVIDENCE-BASED DESIGN AND BEST PRACTICES"

Decades of empirical research substantiate that thoughtfully designed healthcare environments exert a significant influence on patient outcomes. The incorporation of elements such as open spaces, nature-inspired aesthetics, and adaptable patient rooms has been correlated with reductions in aggression, decreased stress levels, and accelerated recovery times. Adherence to evidence-based design principles ensures that facilities are both functionally efficacious and therapeutically advantageous.

CASE STUDY: ARCHITECTURAL BEST PRACTICES AT VCBR

The Virginia Center for Behavioral Rehabilitation (VCBR) implemented architectural best practices to enhance resident and staff safety and improve treatment outcomes. This initiative exemplifies how evidence-based design can transform behavioral health facilities into environments that foster well-being and rehabilitation.

Commitment to Lifelong Learning

The dynamic nature of behavioral healthcare necessitates a commitment to continuous professional development. Practitioners must remain abreast of advancements in treatment methodologies, regulatory amendments, and design innovations. Active participation in professional organizations, attendance at industry conferences, and analysis of real-world case studies are vital practices that ensure teams maintain a position at the vanguard of the industry.

Insight: Centre for Addiction and Mental Health (CAMH)

At CAMH, the establishment of a Project Management Office (PMO) and the provision of internal professional development opportunities have been instrumental. Team members engage in brainstorming sessions and educational courses encompassing topics such as "presentation skills" and "change management," cultivating a culture of continuous improvement.

THE POWER OF TEAMWORK: COLLABORATIVE ENGAGEMENT

The development of behavioral health facilities is strongest when built on **collaborative engagement** -where each stakeholder contributes unique expertise toward a shared vision.

Inclusive Decision-Making & Cross-Disciplinary Collaboration

What It Is: Involving clinical staff, operational leaders, security experts, patients, and community representatives in the design and planning process.

Why It Matters:

- Anticipates operational and cultural challenges.
- Generates innovative, real-world solutions.
- Builds alignment between design and care delivery.

Shared Accountability & Project Transparency

What It Is: Establishing clear roles, responsibilities, and communication protocols.

Why It Matters:

- Promotes trust across the team.
- Keeps all disciplines aligned with the mission.
- Reduces conflict and ambiguity during execution.

Insight – Integrated Project Delivery (IPD):

Case studies demonstrate that projects using IPD achieve higher efficiency and innovation by fostering transparency, delineated responsibilities, and shared accountability among all parties.

Stakeholder Support & Community Endorsement

The success of behavioral health facilities is inseparable from **community acceptance and trust**.

Building Community Trust:

- Address stigma and misconceptions proactively.
- Educate the public on the value of behavioral health facilities.
- Share stories of impact to humanize the mission.

Stakeholder Involvement in Planning:

- Engage local officials, healthcare providers, and advocacy groups early.
- Align project goals with community needs.
- Expedite approvals by demonstrating collaborative intent.

Insight – Change Management in Healthcare Planning:

Studies show that projects incorporating stakeholder involvement into project management frameworks achieve more effective and widely accepted outcomes.

Full-Cycle Coordination Excellence

Seamless coordination across **all project phases** -from planning to occupancy -is essential to minimize delays, control costs, and maximize performance.

Technology-Driven Project Management:

- Employ digital platforms such as **Building Information Modeling (BIM), Procore, or Primavera P6**.

- Monitor progress in real time.
- Anticipate and address bottlenecks before they become critical.
- Centralize information for all disciplines, ensuring consistent communication and reducing misalignment.

KEY TAKEAWAY

Behavioral health facility development succeeds when **collaborative teamwork, community trust, and precise coordination** work in harmony. By combining **inclusive decision-making, shared accountability, proactive stakeholder engagement, and technology-driven management**, teams create facilities that are not only compliant and efficient but also **trusted sanctuaries of healing**.

CASE STUDY: CENTRE FOR ADDICTION AND MENTAL HEALTH (CAMH), TORONTO

The CAMH Queen Street redevelopment in Toronto, one of Canada's most substantial transformations of a mental health hospital, utilized BIM technology to integrate disparate project components. By leveraging real-time digital modeling, the team obviated clashes between structural, mechanical, and electrical systems prior to construction, thus minimizing costly mid-project modifications. This technology-driven approach enabled CAMH to inaugurate a state-of-the-art mental health center that integrates therapeutic environments with operational efficiency.

CLEAR ROLE DEFINITIONS AND ACCOUNTABILITY

Absent precise delineation of responsibilities, even optimally funded projects may descend into disarray. The Design-Build Institute of America (DBIA) underscores the significance of well-defined roles, particularly in Integrated Project Delivery (IPD) and Design-Build models. Owners' Advisors fulfill a crucial role in aligning architects, engineers, and contractors to a unified vision, ensuring that directives from leadership are accurately translated to the construction site.

CASE STUDY: VENTURA COUNTY MEDICAL CENTER

When Ventura County Medical Center necessitated a new mental health facility, the preliminary definition of roles was paramount. The Owner's Advisor facilitated the creation of a Project Charter, delineating each participant's responsibilities, deliverables, and performance metrics. This framework precluded scope creep, augmented contractor accountability, and ensured stakeholder alignment, culminating in on-time, on-budget completion without significant change orders.

RISK MANAGEMENT: CONTINGENCY PLANNING

Unforeseen challenges, ranging from material shortages to regulatory hurdles, are an inherent aspect of complex projects. Proactive risk mitigation initiates with comprehensive risk assessments that identify potential obstacles before they escalate into critical crises. An Owner's Advisor, drawing upon extensive experience, can discern latent risks, such as unanticipated site conditions, evolving health code mandates, or modifications in reimbursement structures for behavioral health services. By incorporating contingency planning and phased budgeting, the project team can adapt promptly when disruptions occur.

CASE STUDY: BEHAVIORAL HEALTH FACILITY IN FLORIDA

A major behavioral health center in Florida encountered a sudden state funding reallocation, jeopardizing project completion. Through the pre-identification of alternative funding sources, including private donations and municipal bonds, the project maintained solvency and was inaugurated as scheduled. This degree of financial foresight is a hallmark of Owner's Advisors, ensuring that mission-critical facilities are not imperiled by unforeseen circumstances.

THE ROLE OF EXPERIENCED OWNER'S ADVISORS: EXPERT GUIDANCE

> "If you want to go fast, go alone. If you want to go far, go together."
>
> AFRICAN PROVERB

Developing a behavioral health facility is among the most complex challenges in real estate. Unlike office buildings or retail centers, these projects must integrate **clinical, therapeutic, and security considerations** while navigating **strict regulatory frameworks**. The presence of a seasoned **Owner's Advisor** often determines whether a project thrives -or fails.

STRATEGIC ALIGNMENT: BEYOND CONSULTING

An Owner's Advisor is not a detached consultant but an **embedded advocate** who safeguards the project's mission. They guide stakeholders through critical questions and decisions:

- **Project Goals & Vision** – Is the facility designed for crisis stabilization, long-term treatment, or outpatient care?
- **Clinical & Operational Needs** – What patient capacity, room types, and security measures are required?
- **Regulatory & Compliance Requirements** – How do shifting behavioral health policies shape design and approval?

⚠️ Without this guidance, organizations risk "scope drift," where incremental design changes undermine the core mission and leave the facility unable to meet its intended purpose.

FINANCIAL ACUMEN: CONTROLLING COSTS WITHOUT COMPROMISE

Behavioral health projects typically operate on **thin margins**. Budget overruns during development can weaken future service delivery. An Owner's Advisor brings **financial expertise** to ensure resources are maximized:

- **Federal & State Grants** – Medicaid initiatives, HUD programs, and behavioral health infrastructure funds.
- **Public-Private Partnerships (P3s)** – Leveraging private capital to offset upfront costs.
- **Phased Construction Financing** – Spreading expenditures across funding cycles for sustainability.

Case Insight – California Behavioral Health Campus:

When a large California project faced spiraling construction costs, the Owner's Advisor restructured financing through a **P3 model**, securing **$15M in additional funding**. This preserved design integrity while keeping the project solvent.

ADVOCACY FOR INNOVATION & BEST PRACTICES

Owner's Advisors ensure facilities are **built for tomorrow, not just today**. They promote forward-thinking strategies such as:

- **Biophilic Design** – Natural light, green spaces, and organic textures to reduce stress and promote healing.
- **Deinstitutionalized Aesthetics** – Calming, home-like interiors that replace cold institutional environments.
- **Smart Technology Integration** – Patient monitoring systems that enhance safety while maintaining dignity and privacy.

TOP 10 RESPONSIBILITIES OF OWNER'S ADVISORS

1. **Mission Alignment**
   - Protect the project's vision, goals, and purpose.
   - Prevent "scope drift" that dilutes core objectives.
2. **Stakeholder Coordination**
   - Align Owner, design, finance, clinical, and community voices.
   - Resolve conflicts early and maintain communication flow.
3. **Regulatory Navigation**
   - Ensure compliance with licensing, zoning, building codes, and healthcare regulations.
   - Anticipate policy changes that affect design or operations.
4. **Budget Oversight**
   - Monitor costs continuously.
   - Identify opportunities for grants, tax credits, and P3 financing.
5. **Schedule Management**
   - Align funding cycles with permitting deadlines.
   - Ensure construction milestones integrate with clinical activation.
6. **Risk Mitigation**
   - Conduct risk assessments across structural, legal, environmental, and financial domains.
   - Secure proper insurance coverage and contingency planning.
7. **Quality Assurance**
   - Uphold clinical, therapeutic, and safety standards.
   - Integrate trauma-informed and healing-centered design.
8. **Innovation Advocacy**
   - Champion biophilic design, deinstitutionalized aesthetics, and smart technology integration.
   - Future-proof facilities against evolving clinical needs.
9. **Community Engagement**
   - Build public trust through transparency.
   - Involve local stakeholders to reduce opposition and accelerate approvals.

10. **Operational Readiness**
    - Ensure workflows, staffing, and clinical models are integrated into facility design.
    - Transition the project seamlessly from construction to active care.

KEY SUCCESS FACTORS OF OWNER'S ADVISOR

- Early and consistent **involvement** across all phases.
- **Neutrality**: Advocates for the Owner, not vendors or contractors.
- **Documentation discipline**: Every decision tracked, every risk logged.
- **High-trust leadership**: Builds cohesion and maintains accountability.

KEY TAKEAWAY

A skilled Owner's Advisor is the **strategic glue** in behavioral health development. They align stakeholders, protect the mission, manage financial risks, and advocate for future-ready design. With their expertise, organizations can avoid costly missteps and deliver facilities that are **sustainable, compliant, innovative, and truly healing**.

> "The best teamwork comes from men who are working independently toward one goal in unison."
>
> JAMES CASH PENNEY

FRONT LINE STORY #25. "TEAMWORK TRIUMPH"

We were six months away from opening a new facility when we hit a perfect storm of problems. A critical shipment of specialized flooring was delayed by two months due to a supply chain issue, a city inspector raised a last-minute, unexpected concern about our fire suppression system, and a key funding reimbursement was held up by a bureaucratic error. Any one of these issues could have delayed our opening; all three at once felt catastrophic. Panic was setting in.

Instead of pointing fingers, the project leadership team held an emergency all-hands-on-deck meeting. It was a moment of true teamwork. The general contractor immediately re-sequenced the interior work, shifting crews to areas that didn't require the delayed flooring, which kept his team productive and on-site. Our architect, who had a long-standing relationship with the city, met directly with the fire marshal to understand his concerns, and together they developed a minor, low-cost modification that satisfied the requirement without a formal redesign. Meanwhile, as the Owner's Advisor, I worked with our financial manager to provide the funding agency with the precise documentation needed to resolve their error and release the funds. We overcame a potential three-month delay in just two weeks because every member of the team trusted each other, took ownership of their piece of the puzzle, and worked in unison toward the same goal: getting the doors open for the community that needed us.

SUMMARY: THE MISSING KEY – THE OWNER'S ADVISOR

> "An investment in knowledge pays the best interest."
>
> BENJAMIN FRANKLIN

Developing behavioral health facilities is not merely about constructing buildings - it is about creating environments that heal. Every choice, from site selection to furniture placement, shapes patient outcomes, staff efficiency, and community integration.

Excellence requires:

- **Rigorous Quality Standards**
- Grounded in evidence-based design, clinical insight, and proven case studies.
- **Interdisciplinary Collaboration**
- Integrating architects, engineers, clinicians, operators, and community voices.

- **Stakeholder Engagement**
- Building public trust and ensuring facilities serve long-term community needs.
- **Seamless Coordination**
- Utilizing technology, structured project management, and real-time communication to prevent delays and inefficiencies.
- **The Experienced Owner's Advisor**
- The missing key -a trusted advocate who aligns vision, safeguards mission, and ensures that projects deliver not just a facility, but a sanctuary for recovery.

FINAL THOUGHT: A CALL TO ACTION

Behavioral health development is a mission-driven endeavor. It requires visionary leadership, unwavering commitment, and expert guidance. The Owner's Advisor is the anchor: the strategist, advocate, and problem-solver who transforms blueprints into healing spaces. By embracing the principles outlined in this chapter, we can create behavioral health facilities that are not just buildings but lifelines for those in need. As we move forward, let us remember, "The best way to predict the future is to create it." With the right expertise and dedication, we can build a future where every individual has access to the behavioral health support they deserve.

PART FOUR
PERMITTING, CONSTRUCTION & CLOSEOUT

Chapter 15

Procurement and PRECONSTRUCTION

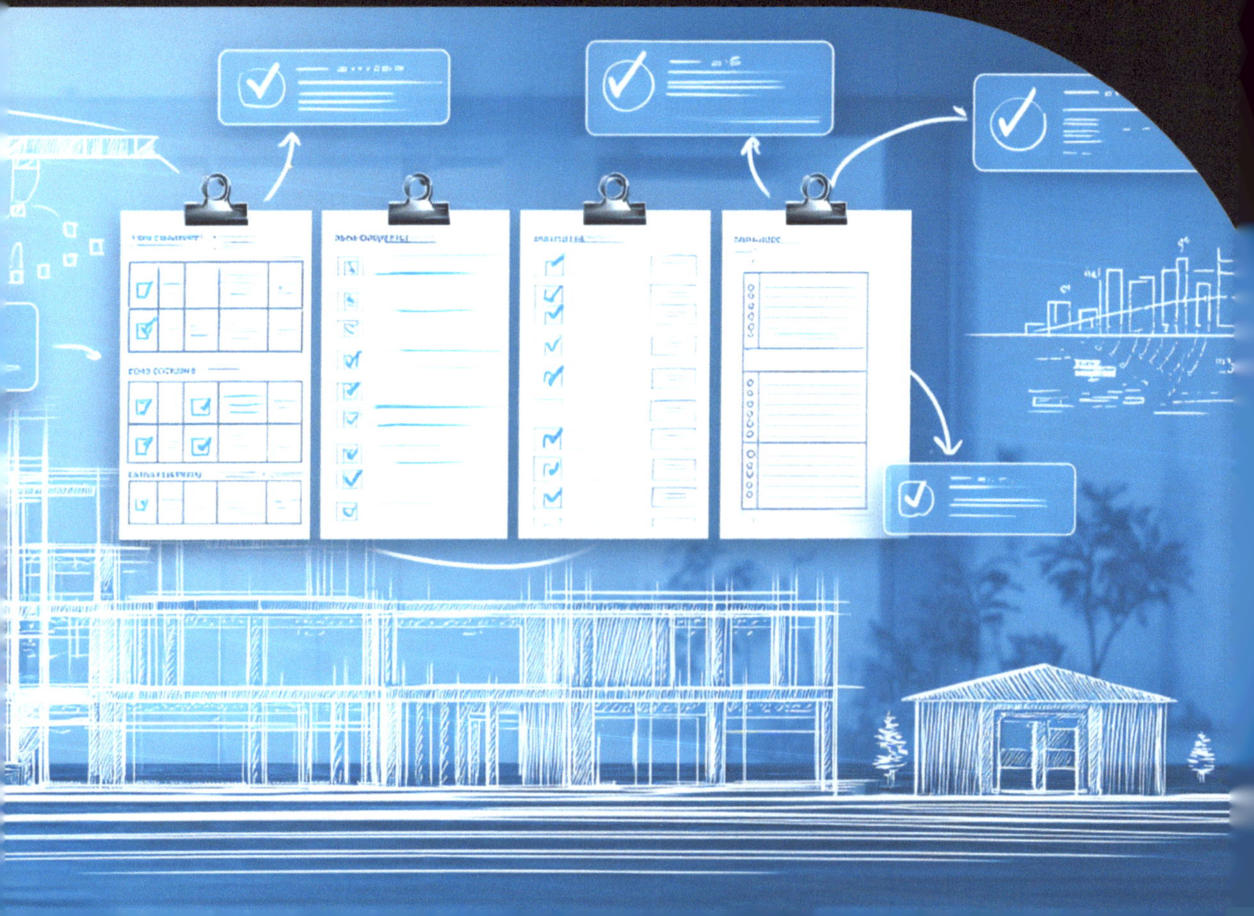

CHAPTER 15
PROCUREMENT AND PRECONSTRUCTION

WHAT YOU'LL LEARN:

1. Value Engineering with Purpose
2. GMP Negotiations and Bid Leveling Strategies
3. Vendor and Specialty Consultant Procurement
4. Managing Procurement Timelines in Rapid Delivery Models
5. Ensuring Scope Clarity to Prevent Change Orders

> "Plans are nothing; planning is everything."
>
> DWIGHT D. EISENHOWER

CHAPTER PURPOSE

This chapter demystifies the pivotal transition from planning to physical execution. Procurement and pre-construction are where your project's vision becomes a quantifiable strategy. For behavioral health developments, where every dollar matters and every detail impacts vulnerable populations, this stage is not just preparatory; it's foundational.

Accurate thinking makes procurement and preconstruction strategic, not just procedural. Compare like with like, name assumptions, and decide with evidence. In behavioral health, clarity in scope and pricing prevents downstream change and protects trust.

Operationalize with a scoring matrix, interview rubric, and bid-leveling workbook. Publish alternates and exclusions early. Run constructability and value sessions that improve the documents before locking price. Confirm long-lead items and logistics so the plan is buildable.

FRONT LINE STORY # 26. VALUE ENGINEERING WITH PURPOSE

> "The bitterness of poor quality remains long after the sweetness of low price is forgotten."
>
> BENJAMIN FRANKLIN

We were in the final stages of budgeting for a new community wellness center, and the initial bids came in nearly 15% over our budget. The immediate suggestion from the contractor was to cut one of the "non-essential" spaces: a large, multipurpose room designed for yoga, art therapy, and community meetings. From a purely financial perspective, it was the easiest cut to make. From a mission perspective, it was unthinkable; that room was the heart of the facility.

Instead of cutting scope, we initiated a value engineering workshop with a clear directive: protect the mission at all costs. The team rose to the challenge. Our interior designer found a different brand of resilient flooring that had the same durability and aesthetic at a 20% cost savings. The architect identified a high-quality, pre-fabricated modular casework system that could replace the custom-milled cabinetry, saving over $100,000 without sacrificing function. By making a series of these intelligent, targeted substitutions, we were able to bring the project back on budget without eliminating a single square foot of programmable space. It was a powerful lesson that "value engineering" isn't about making a project cheaper; it's about making it smarter.

Section 1: Value Engineering with Purpose

> "Value engineering is not about cutting costs; it's about maximizing impact with the dollars you have."
>
> OWNER

Core Principles

- Align all cost-reduction efforts with the patient-centered mission
- Maintain performance, safety, and design intent
- Evaluate long-term facility operation and maintenance impacts

Structured VE Process

- Define Scope & Intent: Set VE goals and constraints upfront
- Host VE Workshops: Involve interdisciplinary stakeholders
- Use Decision Logs: Document choices and rationale
- Evaluate Risk: Vet tradeoffs with lifecycle performance metrics

Practical Applications

Element	VE Opportunity	Benefit
Lighting	Smart LED systems	Energy savings, staff comfort
Casework	Modular, standardized designs	Lower installation cost
Exterior Finishes	Fiber cement over masonry	Cost and aesthetic retention
Flooring	Resilient sheet vs. LVT	Infection control and value

Section 2: GMP Negotiations and Bid Leveling Strategies

"You don't get what you deserve; you get what you negotiate."

CHESTER L. KARRASS

GMP Must-Haves

- Detailed line-item breakdowns
- Transparent general conditions and fees
- Allowances and contingency controls
- Clear owner-directed alternates and assumptions

Best Practices for Bid Leveling

- Create a Bid Comparison Matrix
- Interview subs for clarification
- Require breakout pricing and unit rates
- Reconcile bid exclusions through Addenda or RFIs

Owner's Advisor Tools

- Pre-negotiation checklist
- GMP risk register
- Joint scope review templates

Section 3: Vendor and Specialty Consultant Procurement

"You're only as strong as your weakest subcontractor."

INDUSTRY CLICHÉ

Specialized Vendors for Behavioral Health

- FF&E with ligature resistance
- Low-voltage integrators
- Nurse call and duress systems
- Behavioral safety signage and controls

Evaluation Criteria

Factor	Weight (%)	Considerations
Relevant Experience	30%	Similar healthcare/behavioral projects
Compliance Readiness	25%	ICRA, ADA, HIPAA, OSHPD standards
Cost Competitiveness	20%	Transparent pricing, detailed inclusions
Technical Innovation	15%	Tech stack, installation lead time, compatibility
Financial Strength	10%	Insurance, bonding, history

Pro Tips

- Always cross-check vendor assumptions with drawings and narratives
- Build a prequalified vendor pool for time-sensitive scopes
- Use a procurement specialist to manage solicitations and Q&A

Section 4: Managing Procurement Timelines in Rapid Delivery Models

> "What gets measured gets managed."
>
> PETER DRUCKER

Key Concepts

- Procurement influences the critical path more than design
- Lead-time variability drives risk on aggressive schedules

Tools for Timeline Management

- Procurement Gantt Chart: Align vendor buyouts with trade mobilization
- Submittal Tracker: Ensure early approval of shop drawings
- Weekly Logistics Reviews: Monitor product delivery and fabrication

Behavioral Health Long-Lead Examples

Equipment	Lead Time	Risk Mitigation Strategy
Ligature-Resistant Fixtures (sample approval required)	16–24 weeks	Order with DD drawings
RTLS Systems	12–20 weeks	Coordinate with IT and electrical design
Specialized HVAC Units	20+ weeks	Issue as early procurement package

Section 5: Ensuring Scope Clarity to Prevent Change Orders

> "Clarity is kindness."
>
> BRENÉ BROWN

Clarity Measures

- Conduct page-turn workshops with the Owner, CM, and Design team
- Issue a Room-by-Room Matrix with detailed responsibilities
- Create a trade scope master list with all interdependencies

Preventative Change Order Protocols

- Implement a Pre-GMP Change Order Log
- Host Scope Clarification Workshops for each major package
- Track every owner decision and scope freeze deadline
- Create a "No Surprises" pledge within your project charter

> "The single biggest problem in communication is the illusion that it has taken place."
>
> GEORGE BERNARD SHAW

FRONT LINE STORY #27. CLARITY IN SCOPE

Before signing a Guaranteed Maximum Price (GMP) contract with our general contractor, I insisted on a series of "scope alignment" meetings with their key subcontractors. It felt like a tedious, time-consuming step, but my experience told me it was crucial. During the meeting with the electrical subcontractor, we did a page turn of the drawings for the nurse call system.

The subcontractor pointed to a note on the plans and said, "This is a bit ambiguous. We are assuming the wiring needs to be run in a standard conduit, but if it requires a plenum-rated, low-smoke conduit because of the HVAC system design, that's a $150,000 cost difference." The room went quiet. The MEP engineer and the architect quickly confirmed that the higher-rated conduit was indeed required. By having that conversation before the GMP was signed, we were able to include the correct cost in the contract. Had we not, that ambiguity would have resulted in a massive, unavoidable change order halfway through the project. That one meeting saved the project from a major budget crisis and reinforced a core principle: clarity up front is the most effective form of risk management.

CHAPTER SUMMARY: PROCUREMENT AS STRATEGIC EXECUTION

Procurement and preconstruction set the tone for construction. Done well, they eliminate chaos, reduce uncertainty, and enhance team confidence. Done poorly, they breed conflict, cost overruns, and delays. This stage isn't about pushing paper; it's about project leadership. The Owner's Advisor, working in tandem with designers, contractors, and vendors, becomes the thread that weaves all complexity into clarity.

Leadership Insight: "In real estate, execution is everything. But before that, it's alignment."

In the chapters to come, we shift from planning to action, where the quality of your preconstruction preparation will be tested on every beam, wall, and system installed in the field.

Chapter 16

Construction Management and Field **OVERSIGHT**

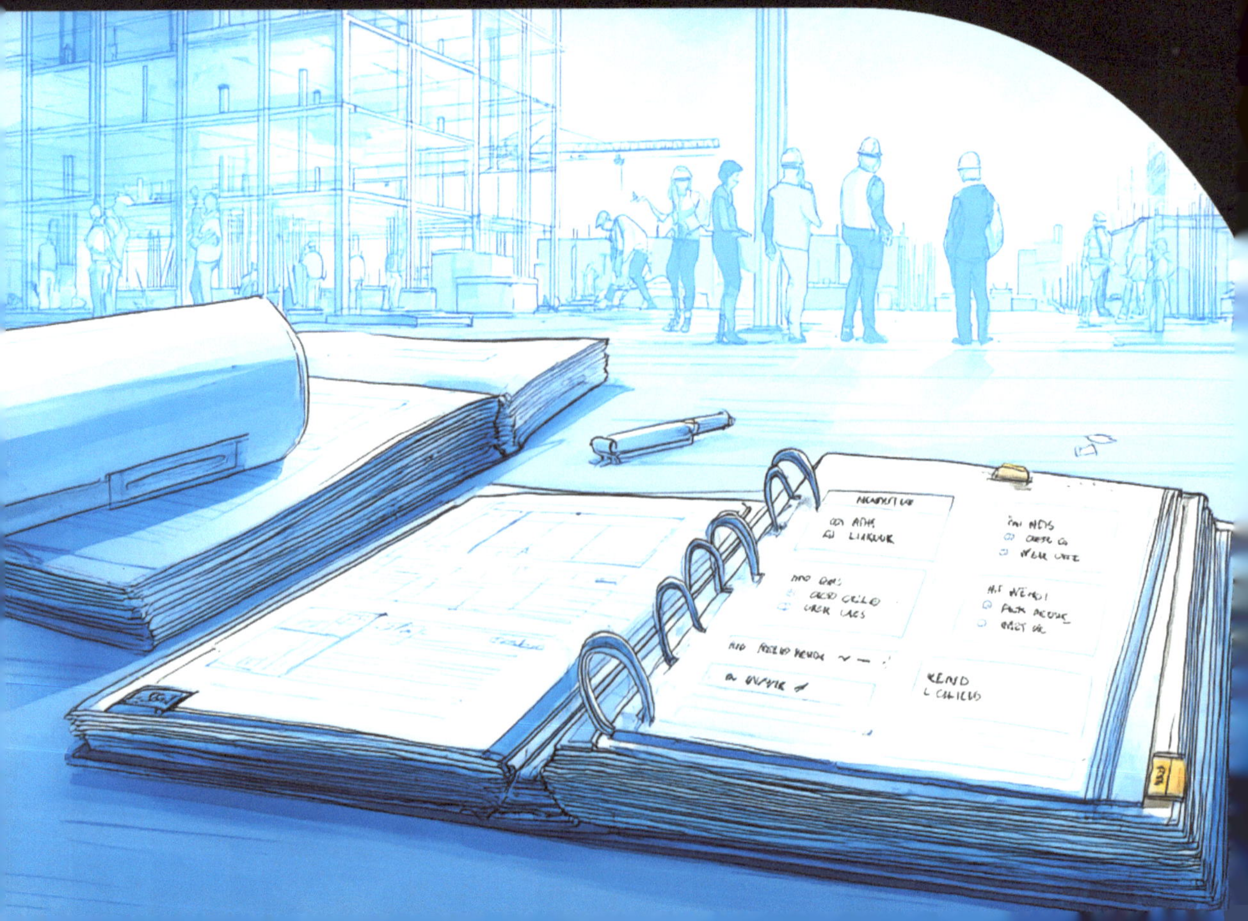

CHAPTER 16
CONSTRUCTION MANAGEMENT AND FIELD OVERSIGHT

WHAT YOU WILL LEARN IN THIS CHAPTER:

- Managing Construction with Behavioral Health Complexity in Mind
- Weekly Field Coordination and Look-Ahead Scheduling
- RFI and Submittal Processes Optimized for Rapid Delivery
- Managing Quality, Safety, Inspections, and Milestone Tracking
- Documenting Progress and Avoiding Litigation Traps

CHAPTER OVERVIEW

Construction is where vision meets reality, and where leadership, coordination, and documentation must be executed with precision and discipline. In behavioral health real estate projects, the construction phase is especially sensitive due to high regulatory scrutiny, complex operational needs, and the vulnerability of future occupants.

This chapter provides a framework of field-tested strategies and DBIA-backed best practices for managing behavioral health construction, emphasizing the vital role of the Owner's Advisor in steering the project to completion.

Persistence and self-control keep construction aligned with intent when the field gets noisy. Stay calm, clear, and consistent. Protect the therapeutic goals while solving problems in sequence.

Run construction with disciplined oversight. Hold weekly quality walks, manage RFIs and submittals to rhythm, and maintain a change log that keeps scope under control. Use lookahead schedules and daily huddles so crews see what success looks like before they start. Capture and assign at least ten observations weekly with clear owners.

KEY AREAS OF FOCUS IN BEHAVIORAL HEALTH CONSTRUCTION

1. Managing Construction with Behavioral Health Complexity

Behavioral health facilities demand heightened technical rigor. Ligature resistance, infection control, dual inspections, and secured zones require **early coordination** between architects, engineers, and clinical leads.

Owner's Advisor Role: Enforces compliance and clinical compatibility - preventing costly redesigns or rework.

2. Weekly Field Coordination & Look-Ahead Scheduling

DBIA research shows structured look-ahead meetings make projects **45% more likely** to meet milestones.

- Trade sequencing, inspection prep, and recovery planning must be addressed weekly.
- Look-ahead schedules should be **tracked and enforced** by the Owner's Advisor.

3. Optimizing RFI & Submittal Processes

Critical path issues must not stall progress.

- RFIs/submittals follow a **tiered escalation model** with 48-hour resolution targets.
- Use **real-time dashboards** and milestone crosswalks to minimize procurement delays.
- A **clear chain of accountability** ensures rapid issue resolution.

4. Quality, Safety, & Inspection Readiness

Precision planning is essential to meet regulatory standards.

- Weekly toolbox talks, punchlists, and readiness checklists.
- ICRA adherence and milestone walkthroughs aligned with licensing.
- **Owner's Advisor Role:** Verifies inspection readiness, logs issues, and drives closure.

5. Coordination with HCAI Inspector of Record (IOR) & Licensing Agencies

The IOR functions as the **regulatory gatekeeper**.

- Build relationships early, provide transparent updates, and hold shared readiness walkthroughs.
- **Owner's Advisor Role:** Acts as translator between field teams and agencies, ensuring expectations are met and approvals streamlined.

6. Documentation & Litigation Risk Avoidance

Strong documentation is both compliance and protection.

- Digital logs, field reports, photographic records, and issue trackers.
- Biweekly audits by the Owner's Advisor to ensure consistency across agencies.
- **Result:** Reduced disputes, minimized liability, and airtight compliance.

✅ When applied consistently, these practices transform complex behavioral health projects into predictable, compliant, and successful outcomes.

✅ QUICK REFERENCE CHECKLIST

Behavioral Health Construction – Key Focus Areas for Owners' Advisors

🏗️ 1. Managing Construction with Behavioral Health Complexity

☐ Confirm ligature-resistant and infection-control features.
☐ Coordinate secured patient & staff zones early with A/E team.
☐ Verify design compatibility with clinical and regulatory needs.

📅 2. Weekly Field Coordination & Look-Ahead Scheduling

☐ Hold weekly look-ahead meetings with all trades.
☐ Track sequencing, inspections, and recovery plans.
☐ Document milestones and update owners weekly.

📁 3. RFI & Submittal Process Optimization

☐ Enforce 48-hour resolution target for critical RFIs/submittals.
☐ Use dashboard tracking for status and bottlenecks.
☐ Maintain clear accountability chain for issue resolution.

🛠️ 4. Quality, Safety & Inspection Readiness

☐ Conduct weekly toolbox talks & punchlist reviews.
☐ Align ICRA and safety measures with milestones.
☐ Verify readiness before each inspection with checklists.

🏛️ 5. Coordination with HCAI IOR & Licensing Agencies

☐ Build relationship early with IOR & regulators.
☐ Share transparent updates and readiness walkthroughs.
☐ Translate field conditions into compliance language.

6. Documentation & Litigation Risk Mitigation

- ☐ Maintain daily digital logs and photo documentation.
- ☐ Track issues and resolutions in real time.
- ☐ Perform biweekly documentation audits for compliance.

Advisor's Role

- Enforce **discipline in coordination**.
- Act as **compliance translator**.
- Ensure **quality + financial sustainability** through structured oversight.

> "Details create the big picture."
>
> SANFORD I. WEILL

FRONT LINE STORY #28. MANAGING COMPLEXITY

During the construction of an inpatient psychiatric unit, our team had to install specialized anti-ligature fixtures in all patient bathrooms to ensure safety. The plumbing subcontractor, though skilled, had never worked in a behavioral health setting before. During his daily walkthrough, our site superintendent, who had been trained on the project's specific safety requirements, noticed that standard fixtures were being installed out of habit.

He immediately but respectfully stopped the work. Instead of simply issuing a correction notice, we saw it as a critical teaching moment. The Owner's Advisor, the superintendent, and a clinical representative facilitated hands-on training for the entire plumbing crew right there on site. Using a mock-up room, they demonstrated the correct installation process for the anti-ligature hardware and explained why it was a life-or-death detail. This proactive oversight and education didn't just prevent a major safety risk and the costly rework of two dozen rooms; it empowered the trade partner with new expertise and reinforced our team's shared commitment to patient safety.

BEST PRACTICES IN BEHAVIORAL HEALTH CONSTRUCTION

(Owner's Advisor Quick Reference)

1. MANAGING CONSTRUCTION WITH BEHAVIORAL HEALTH COMPLEXITY

Behavioral health construction is not conventional. It requires:

- Ligature-resistant hardware & tamper-proof components
- Seismic anchoring for safety-rated furniture
- Class III/IV infection control (ICRA compliance)
- Secure observation corridors & staff retreat zones
- Dual inspections (fire + licensing)

✅ **Best Practice:** Maintain a Behavioral Health Construction Compliance Checklist at each milestone.

2. WEEKLY FIELD COORDINATION & LOOK-AHEAD SCHEDULING

> "The key is not to prioritize what's on your schedule, but to schedule your priorities."
>
> STEPHEN COVEY

DBIA (2022): Projects with weekly field coordination are **45% more likely** to meet milestones.

Three-Week Look-Ahead Planning

Week	Lead Role	Focus
1	Superintendent	Site logistics, staging, major trades
2	Project Manager	Punchlist prep, inspection alignment
3	QA/QC Foreman	RFI clearance, long-lead review

Pull Planning Tips:

- Sticky-note scheduling with color codes
- Assign leads/dates to resolve blockers
- Align trades on access, inspections, and sequence

Owner's Advisor Role: Monitor adherence, flag risks early, recommend recovery steps.

3. RFI & SUBMITTAL PROCESSES OPTIMIZED FOR RAPID DELIVERY

DBIA (2023): Clear RFI/submittal workflows cut change orders **by 50%.**

Submittal Workflow: Submittal → Design Review (3–5 days) → Return to GC → Procurement → Install

RFI Prioritization:

- **Tier 1 (Critical Path):** 48 hr turnaround
- **Tier 2 (Design Clarification):** 3–5 days
- **Tier 3 (Documentation Only):** 7–10 days

Owner's Advisor Tools:

- Submittal log with live status

- RFI dashboard with escalation notes
- Milestone mapping for dependencies

4. MANAGING QUALITY, SAFETY & INSPECTIONS

Field Safety Protocols

Focus Area	Frequency	Lead Role	Tool
Toolbox Talks	Daily	GC Site Super	Field Safety Log
Safety Audit	Weekly	GC + Owner Rep	Checklist Form
ICRA Protocols	Daily	ICRA Monitor	Entry Logs

QA/QC Workflow

Substrate Inspection → Rough-In QA → First-in-Place Review → Inspector Sign-Off → Punchlist Turnover

Sample Inspection Calendar

Date	Type	Inspector	Area	Status
May 2	Fire Rough	FM	East Wing	Scheduled
May 4	Med Gas Cert	State	Central Core	In Review
May 7	ADA Ramp Final	Local	Entry Vestibule	Complete

5. COORDINATION WITH HCAI INSPECTOR OF RECORD (IOR)

The IOR is the **regulatory gatekeeper**.

Best Practices:

- Preconstruction kickoff (IOR + GC + Owner's Advisor)
- Maintain a live log of observations & actions

- Invite IOR to mock-ups & milestone inspections

Risk Mitigation:

- Notify IOR immediately of scope changes
- Foster a proactive, respectful partnership
- Keep RFIs, submittals, updates fully transparent

Owner's Advisor Role: Liaison between IOR & clinical leadership; translate regulations; track closure of issues.

6. DOCUMENTING PROGRESS & LITIGATION AVOIDANCE

Documentation Hierarchy

Daily Logs → Weekly Photos → Field Reports → Inspection Checklists → Issue Logs → Closeout Records

Litigation Readiness Tracker

Type	Frequency	Owner	Platform
RFIs/Responses	Daily	CM + Architect	Procore
Change Directives	As Needed	Owner's Advisor	Egnyte
Inspector Reports	Weekly	CM	SharePoint

Owner's Advisor Best Practices:

- Require written confirmation for all field direction
- Use cloud-based platforms with real-time control
- Perform biweekly documentation audits

📊 CONCLUSION: LEADERSHIP IN THE FIELD

Behavioral health construction is about **precision + empathy + regulatory fluency**.

DBIA (2023) Key Data:

- Early Owner's Advisor involvement → **43% more likely** on-time/on-budget
- Integrated teams → **50% fewer change orders**
- Strong inspection coordination → **30% faster licensure**

Summary Best Practices:

- Engage IOR & regulators early
- Maintain live inspection schedules
- Prioritize HCAI, ADA & licensing milestones
- Use cloud platforms for audits

Risk Mitigation Essentials:

- Validate mock-ups before orders
- Track inspector notes & corrective actions
- Escalate unresolved issues with data
- Document everything: "If it's not written, it didn't happen."

FRONT LINE STORY #29. AVOIDING LITIGATION TRAPS

On a previous project, a contractor had submitted a large, messy claim for delays at the end of the job, using a disorganized stack of emails as "proof." It was a nightmare to refute. Having learned from that experience, I implemented a strict, real-time documentation protocol on our next project using a cloud-based platform like Procore.

Every RFI, every submittal, every field directive, and every meeting minute was logged and tracked. When a subcontractor later tried to claim they were delayed by a late design decision, we were able to pull up the digital record instantly. The log showed their RFI had been answered within 48 hours and that the subcontractor themselves had delayed their own shop drawing submission by three weeks. The claim was immediately dropped. It was a clear lesson that diligent, contemporaneous documentation is not bureaucratic overhead; it is the single best tool for creating accountability and avoiding disputes.

FINAL THOUGHT:

As we transition into the final stages of commissioning and operational handoff, the principles discussed herein underscore the indispensable role of field leadership, documentation, and strategic collaboration. What begins as drawings ends as a sanctuary for healing if done right.

Chapter 17

Construction **ADMINISTRATION** and Owner Engagement

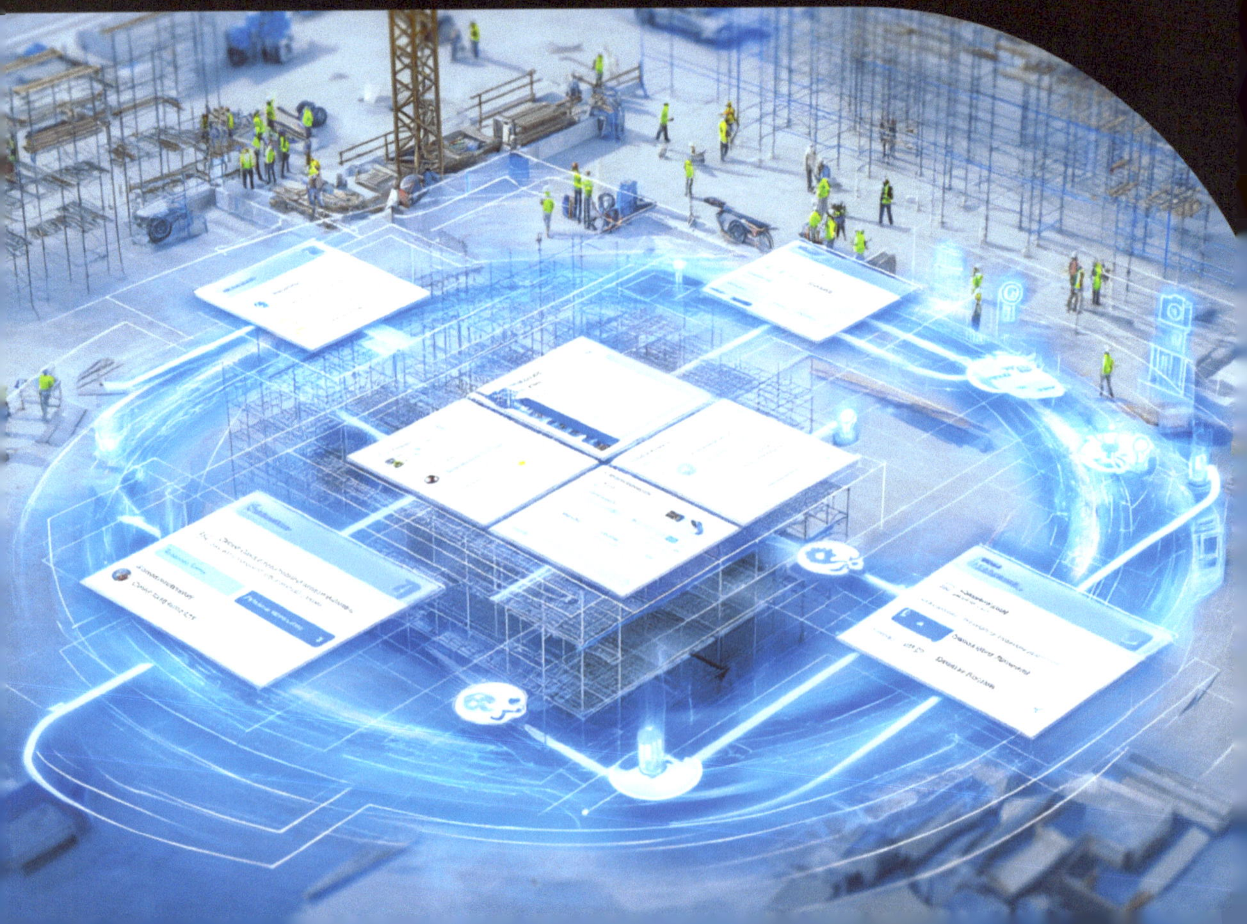

CHAPTER 17
CONSTRUCTION ADMINISTRATION AND OWNER ENGAGEMENT

WHAT YOU WILL LEARN IN THIS CHAPTER:

- Keeping the Owner Informed: Reports, Tours, Decisions
- Field Changes, Change Orders, and Scope Creep Prevention
- Punch Lists, Inspections, and Regulatory Walkthroughs
- Ensuring a Culture of Care During Construction
- Managing Expectations for Substantial Completion

CHAPTER OVERVIEW

Construction administration (CA) represents the critical bridge between field execution and operational activation. It is more than a countdown to completion; it is the time when documentation, inspections, punch lists, and coordination culminate in the final product. For behavioral health facilities, where regulatory scrutiny, clinical precision, and trauma-informed design intersect, this phase must be executed with discipline and integrity.

Accurate thinking and self-control turn construction administration into service. Keep the owner informed, remove friction for the field, and document every decision cleanly. In behavioral health, that steadiness preserves relationships and momentum.

Operationalize with meeting notes that show decisions, action owners, and dates. Maintain a live log of RFIs, COs, and pay apps. Walk the site with curiosity and respect. Close loops daily so surprises shrink.

According to the Design-Build Institute of America (DBIA), projects that engage owners' advisors and implement structured construction administration practices experience 50% fewer change orders, a 36% reduction in final inspection delays, and are 42% more likely to meet budget and schedule targets (DBIA, 2022). Similarly, the American Institute of Architects (AIA) reports that stakeholder-inclusive walkthroughs reduce post-occupancy disruptions by 28% and licensing delays by up to 45% (AIA, 2021).

This chapter outlines best practices, statistics, and proven strategies for successful construction administration and owner engagement. It draws on data from DBIA, AIA, CA DHCS, and field-tested Owner's Advisor experience to ensure smooth turnover, stakeholder confidence, and facility readiness.

FRONT LINE STORY #30. OWNER ENGAGEMENT

On one project, the hospital's CEO was an extremely busy, hands-off leader who preferred to receive updates via a concise weekly email. For months, this system worked well. But as the project moved from structural work to interior finishes, I could sense a growing anxiety. The decisions were becoming more tangible, and the reports, no matter how detailed, weren't providing the CEO with the confidence needed.

Instead of just sending more data, I invited the CEO for a bi-weekly, 30-minute site tour. We put on hard hats and walked the job. I pointed out the progress, explained what was coming next in plain language, and answered questions in the moment. During one of these tours, while walking through a future patient wing, the CEO noticed that the location of a planned hand-sanitizing station would create a minor but annoying workflow issue for the nursing staff. It was a small detail that wasn't apparent on the blueprints but was obvious in person. We were able to relocate it with a simple change order that cost almost nothing. These tours transformed the CEO's anxiety into excitement and ownership. That simple act of open communication and direct engagement didn't just build trust; it made the project better.

KEY AREAS OF FOCUS

Keeping the Owner Informed: Reports, Tours, Decisions

Transparency is essential. Owners must have a clear line of sight into daily progress, budget shifts, schedule risks, and inspection readiness.

Best Practices Include:

- Weekly summary reports with milestone tracking, budget exposure updates, and licensing preparation.
- Regular Owner walkthroughs to monitor field conditions and identify activation needs.
- Live dashboards for RFIs, submittals, and open action items.
- Decision logs tracked by the Owner's Advisor to ensure accountability.

Common Challenges & Solutions:

Overwhelmed Owners: The solution is to assign an Owner's Advisor to interpret technical data and guide decision-making.

Gaps in communication: The solution is to use structured engagement sessions with documentation summaries.

Missed approvals: The solution is to set clear decision deadlines tied to procurement and inspection readiness.

Field Changes, Change Orders, and Scope Creep Prevention

Changes are inevitable but must be tightly controlled. According to DBIA research, projects that use formal change control processes reduce cost overruns by 37% (DBIA, 2021).

Best Practices Include:

- A structured change order workflow with justification, impact review, and written approval.
- Ongoing change tracking through a centralized cost management tool.
- Weekly scope review meetings led by the Owner's Advisor.

COMMON CHALLENGES & SOLUTIONS IN BEHAVIORAL HEALTH FACILITY CONSTRUCTION

1. CLINICAL TEAM CHANGE REQUESTS LATE IN CONSTRUCTION

Challenge: Last-minute clinical requests disrupt cost and schedule.

Solution: Educate stakeholders early on the **financial and schedule impacts** of each change.

2. SCOPE DRIFT

Challenge: Incremental changes erode mission clarity.

Solution: Enforce strict **"scope freeze" checkpoints** at key milestones.

3. BUDGET OVERRUNS

Challenge: Change requests without financial backing derail budgets.

Solution: Require every change request to include an **identified funding source**.

📝 PUNCH LISTS, INSPECTIONS & REGULATORY WALKTHROUGHS

DHCS research: **62% of licensing delays** stem from uncoordinated inspection readiness.

Best Practices

- Begin punchlisting **early** (by floor/zone).
- Involve facilities, nursing, and licensing teams in readiness walks.
- Conduct **mock walkthroughs** with HCAI, Fire Marshal, and DHCS.

Common Challenges & Solutions

- **Missed items** → Use a **punch list app** with photos & responsibility tags.
- **Incomplete inspection docs** → Maintain a **binder per agency** with all required submittals.
- **Scheduling delays** → Keep a **forward-looking inspection calendar**.

🩶 ENSURING A CULTURE OF CARE DURING CONSTRUCTION

AIA Healthcare Design Study (2022): Facilities with contractor training saw**22% higher staff satisfaction** and **17% fewer post-occupancy complaints**.

Best Practices

- Train **all workers** on behavioral health sensitivity.
- Post the **mission statement on-site** and include in subcontractor orientation.
- Hold **regular check-ins** with adjacent departments/early move-in teams.

Common Challenges & Solutions

- **Worker fatigue/disconnection** → Share the **project purpose** and celebrate progress.
- **Disruption of live operations** → Schedule **high-noise work off-hours**.
- **Perception gaps** → Invite **frontline staff** to milestone walkthroughs.

MANAGING EXPECTATIONS FOR SUBSTANTIAL COMPLETION

Substantial completion is not just a date - it is an **operational milestone**.

Best Practices

- Define substantial completion criteria **clearly in the contract**.
- Require **life safety, access control, systems testing, furniture** as prerequisites.
- Use a **commissioning & activation matrix** aligned with licensing.

Common Challenges & Solutions

- **Misaligned expectations** → Develop **shared definitions & checklists** (legal + GC + ops).
- **Uncoordinated move-in** → Engage a **third-party move-in/activation consultant**.
- **Final cleaning/document delays** → Track readiness via **Owner's Advisor-led checklist**.

> "The first rule of any technology used in a business is that automation applied to an efficient operation will magnify the efficiency. The second is that automation applied to an inefficient operation will magnify the inefficiency."
>
> BILL GATES

FRONT LINE STORY #31. SCOPE CREEP PREVENTION

During the construction of a new outpatient clinic, the clinical team was thrilled to see their new space taking shape. Their excitement, however, began to translate into a stream of "small" improvement requests made directly to the site superintendent. A request here for an extra outlet, a request there to move a non-load-bearing wall a few feet. While each request seemed minor and well-intentioned, together they represented significant scope creep that was impacting our budget and schedule.

To manage this, we implemented a formal "Design Enhancement Request" process. We created a simple online form where any team member could submit an idea. The form required a brief justification for the change and an acknowledgment that it would be reviewed against the project's budget, schedule, and mission. This did two things: it provided a structured, respectful channel for ideas, and it encouraged the team to think through the implications of their requests. As the Owner's Advisor, I would review these requests weekly with the project leadership. We even created a "wish list" of approved ideas that we could implement if we found cost savings elsewhere. The process replaced informal, chaotic change with disciplined, transparent decision-making, allowing us to protect the project's commitments while still honoring the team's valuable insights.

"Success in project management lies in anticipating challenges, empowering decision-makers, and leading with clarity and consistency."

PERVASIVE THOUGHT: FINISHING STRONG

Construction administration is where vision becomes reality or falls short. It is the stage where small oversights have large consequences and where leadership, documentation, and follow-through matter most.

OWNER'S ADVISOR IN CONSTRUCTION ADMINISTRATION (CA): THE LAST-MILE LEADER

Key Data Points (DBIA & AIA Research):

- **36% reduction** in final inspection delays when CA protocols are led by an Owner's Advisor.
- **50% fewer change orders** and faster licensure achieved by projects with engaged CA teams (DBIA, 2022).
- **28% fewer post-occupancy disruptions** when clinical stakeholders participate in punchlists.

Insight:

The Owner's Advisor is more than a liaison. They are the **last-mile leader** - tracking details, translating data, coordinating agencies, and keeping the entire team aligned with the project's mission.

In the next chapter, we turn to commissioning and activation, ensuring the facility not only opens but also thrives.

Chapter 18

Commissioning, Closeout and **ACTIVATION**

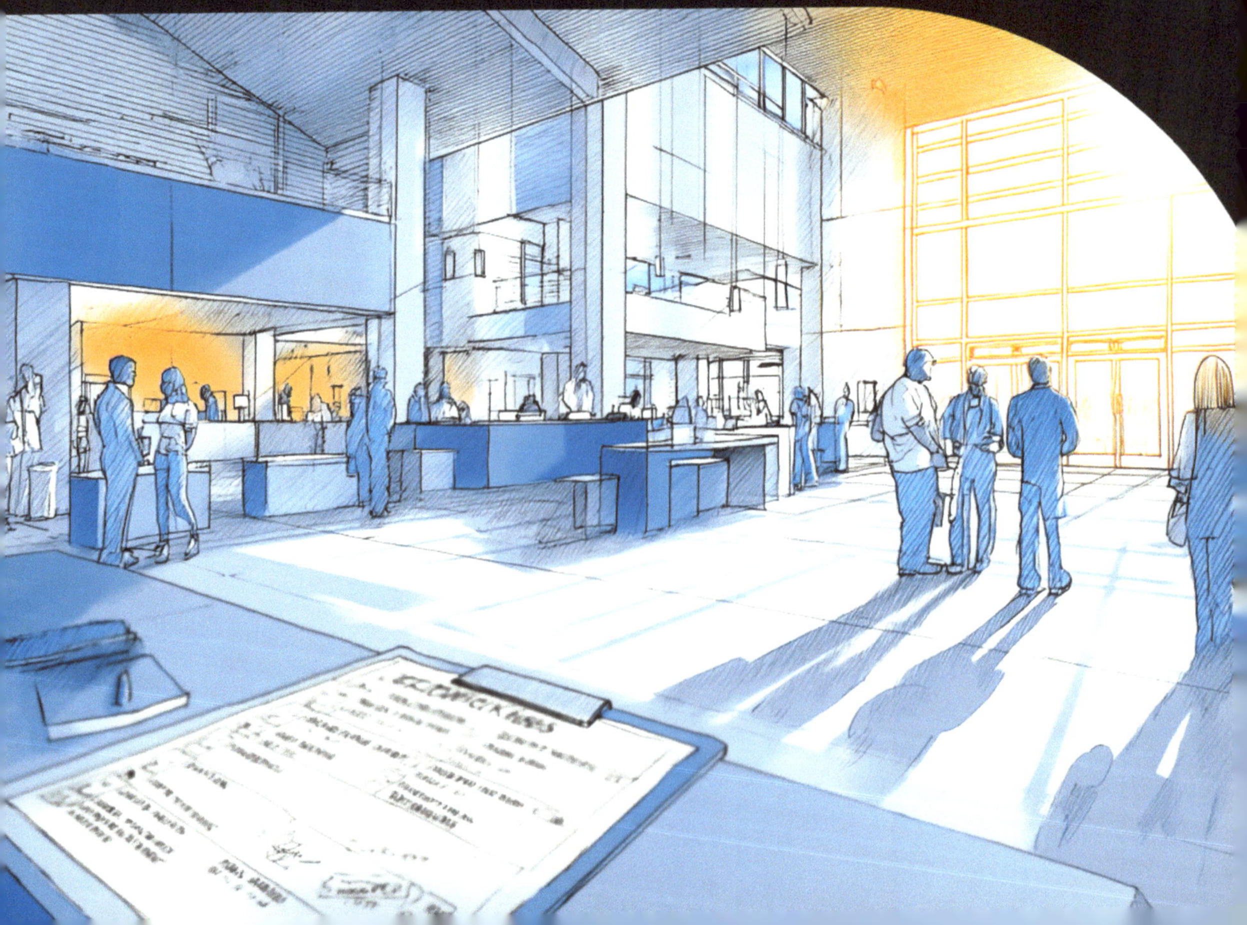

CHAPTER 18
COMMISSIONING, CLOSEOUT, AND ACTIVATION

WHAT YOU WILL LEARN IN THIS CHAPTER:

- Facility Commissioning for Life-Safety and Behavioral Health-Specific Systems
- Transition-to-Operations Planning and Staff Readiness
- O&M Manuals, Training, and Facility Performance
- Managing Warranties, FM Handoff, and 90-Day Tuning
- Lessons Learned and Post-Occupancy Evaluation Strategies

CHAPTER OVERVIEW

This chapter outlines the critical steps, best practices, and field-tested strategies to commission systems, prepare staff, and optimize facility performance. These activities are essential to ensure the building not only opens but also thrives in service to its mission.

Organized planning and persistence finish strong. Pay attention to detail with urgency. In behavioral health, closeout is where safety, training, and dignity meet the first day of care.

Turn mindset into a commissioning and activation checklist that teams can run. Verify systems, train staff, and walk the punch list in order. Publish cutover plans and day-one protocols. Conduct a simulated day-one drill to validate readiness and documentation for regulators and operators.

Commissioning and activation are not the end of the project; they are the beginning of its life. For behavioral health facilities, this phase ensures that buildings not only open but operate seamlessly, safely, and in alignment with the clinical mission. It is a time of testing, training, fine-tuning, and transferring knowledge. Done well, this phase turns handover into healing.

Research from the AIA and DBIA (2022) shows that behavioral health projects with structured commissioning protocols and stakeholder-informed activation plans are 38% more likely to meet operational performance goals within the first 90 days. Furthermore, facilities that conduct post-occupancy evaluations report 25% fewer maintenance issues in year one and a 20% increase in patient and staff satisfaction.

> "You don't close the project. You launch the operation."
>
> PROJECT MANAGEMENT PROVERB

Once the building is occupied, active management of warranties, service calls, and early performance tuning becomes essential to long-term success. This chapter outlines best practices across five critical domains of project closeout.

FRONT LINE STORY #32. SMOOTH TRANSITION TO OPERATIONS

The week before a new children's crisis center was scheduled to open, the building was pristine, all inspections were passed, and the keys were ready to be handed over. But a building is not a business. Instead of just opening the doors, we planned a "Day in the Life" simulation. We brought in the entire clinical and operational staff and ran through a series of mock scenarios: a child arriving in acute distress, a fire drill, a medical emergency, and even a routine shift change.

The simulation was invaluable. The staff quickly realized that the crash cart was stored in a closet that was difficult to access during a mock medical emergency. The nurses found that the workflow in the medication room created a bottleneck when two people tried to access it at once. We even discovered that the Wi-Fi had a dead spot in the family therapy wing. We spent the next three days making small but critical adjustments. When the facility opened to its first real patients, the staff moved with a confidence and coordination that would have been impossible without that simulation. It was a powerful reminder that a smooth opening is not an accident; it's the result of meticulous preparation.

COMMISSIONING, TRANSITION, AND FACILITY READINESS

1. Facility Commissioning for Life Safety & Behavioral Health Systems

Commissioning (Cx) ensures that all systems perform as designed, particularly where **life safety** and **behavioral health-specific needs** overlap (e.g., ligature resistance, negative-pressure rooms, security systems, HVAC zoning, and emergency backup power).

Best Practices

- Engage a certified third-party **Commissioning Agent (CxA)** during design development.
- Create a **Behavioral Health-Specific Commissioning Plan** addressing ligature resistance, airflow, visual monitoring, egress safety, and access control.
- Coordinate testing/validation with **AHJs**: Fire Marshal, Building Inspector, HCAI, DHCS.
- Test critical systems: smoke evacuation, access-controlled doors, backup generators, nurse call stations.

Construction Manager Role

- Align scope with licensing requirements.
- Integrate Cx milestones into the master schedule.
- Lead commissioning meetings, track deficiencies, and close out issues.

Results & Research

- Early Cx planning → **47% higher first-pass life safety inspection success** (DBIA, 2022).
- Commissioned BH facilities → **22% fewer equipment failures** in year one (NIBS, 2021).
- Behavioral health Cx → **15–20% fewer patient safety/comfort complaints** (CHD, 2021).

2. Transition to Operations & Staff Readiness

Operational readiness bridges the gap between a finished building and a functioning care environment.

Best Practices

- Develop a **Transition-to-Operations (T2O) Plan** aligned with commissioning, move-in, and staffing.
- Conduct **"Day-in-the-Life" simulations** to test workflows, emergency responses, and space utilization.
- Create a **Readiness Matrix** mapping tasks across IT, clinical, custodial, and administration.
- Use role-based checklists for each department.

Common Challenges & Solutions

- Incomplete clinical training → Hands-on orientation 4–6 weeks before go-live.

- Miscommunication → Weekly cross-department sync meetings.
- Missed dependencies → Build trackers linking closeout, FF&E, IT, and onboarding.

Results & Research

- Structured T2O → **32% higher staff onboarding satisfaction** (AIA, 2021).
- Simulation-based training → **18% fewer safety events in first 90 days** (Joint Commission, 2022).
- Integrated T2O planning → **28% faster ramp-up to full operations** (HFM Journal, 2022).

3. O&M Manuals, Training, & Facility Performance

Operations & Maintenance documentation underpins long-term performance.

Best Practices

- Provide O&M in **print and searchable digital formats**.
- Host system-specific training by vendors (HVAC, electrical, fire/life safety, BMS).
- Develop an **asset inventory** with preventive maintenance schedules.
- Integrate **analytics dashboards** to monitor performance.

Construction Manager Role

- Verify documentation completeness.
- Record and store training sessions.
- Facilitate structured FM team handoffs.

Results & Research

- Proper FM training → **27% fewer unplanned maintenance costs** in year one (NIBS, 2022).
- Digital O&M systems → **30% faster response times** (Healthcare Facilities Today, 2021).
- Strong handoffs → **22% higher FM staff confidence** (CHD, 2022).

4. Managing Warranties, Handoff & 90-Day Tuning

The first 90 days are critical for tuning systems and resolving latent issues.

Best Practices

- Implement a **90-Day Tuning Plan** for HVAC, lighting, access control.
- Maintain a **Warranty Log** with owners/resolution deadlines.
- Hold joint **Owner–GC–FM walkthroughs** at 30, 60, and 90 days.

Construction Manager Role

- Track open punchlist items tied to warranties.
- Ensure GC accountability for defective/incomplete work.
- Support vendor follow-ups during post-occupancy fine-tuning.

Statistic

- Structured tuning protocols → **35% fewer service calls** in first 6 months (DBIA, 2022).

5. Lessons Learned & Post-Occupancy Evaluation (POE)

Post-occupancy evaluations (POEs) turn experience into continuous improvement.

Best Practices

- Schedule POEs at **6 and 12 months** post-opening.
- Gather feedback via staff surveys and interviews.
- Assess: safety incidents, workflow bottlenecks, energy use, patient feedback.

Implementation

- Document findings in a **Closeout Report**.
- Share insights with future project teams.
- Incorporate results into updated standards.

Results & Research

- Structured POEs → **31% higher likelihood** of effective operational updates and reduced capital repairs in years 2–5 (CHD, 2021).

✅ **Summary:** Commissioning and transition are not technical afterthoughts -they are **strategic processes** that safeguard compliance, empower staff, and deliver patient-centered facilities that perform from day one.

> "The only real mistake is the one from which we learn nothing."
>
> HENRY FORD

FRONT LINE STORY #33. POST-OCCUPANCY INSIGHT

Six months after we completed a new outpatient facility, we conducted a formal Post-Occupancy Evaluation (POE). We surveyed staff and patients and held focus groups to understand what was working and what wasn't. The feedback was overwhelmingly positive, but one consistent issue emerged: while the private therapy rooms were excellent, the large, open-plan central nurse station had become a major source of stress. It was constantly noisy, offered no privacy for sensitive conversations, and created a visual bottleneck.

This single insight became the most important lesson we learned from that project. On our very next facility design, we used that data to completely rethink our approach. Instead of one large, central station, we designed a series of smaller, decentralized "team pods" that were acoustically separated but visually connected to the patient areas. The new design was a resounding success, dramatically improving staff wellness and efficiency. The POE process taught us that a project isn't truly "done" at ribbon-cutting. The real learning begins when the building is alive, and listening to that feedback is the key to continuous improvement.

> "Begin with the end in mind."
>
> STEPHEN R. COVEY

FINAL THOUGHT: "COMMISSIONING WITH PURPOSE"

Commissioning and activation are not just technical milestones; they are moments of mission realization. They define how a facility will serve, protect, and support those who need it most. In behavioral health care, the bar is higher. Systems must function flawlessly, environments must promote recovery, and operations must launch with confidence. The Construction Manager is a pivotal leader in this transition, overseeing closeout activities, enabling the FM team, and ensuring a seamless handoff to operations.

Projects that follow best practices, such as early stakeholder engagement, simulation training, integrated tuning, and structured POEs, experience measurable improvements in safety, satisfaction, and cost efficiency. In the best projects, activation isn't the end; it's the first day of fulfilling the mission. Through rigorous commissioning, clear expectations, and a culture of respect, these facilities don't just open doors; they begin to heal.

Chapter 19

Understanding **BHCIP** Rules and Readiness

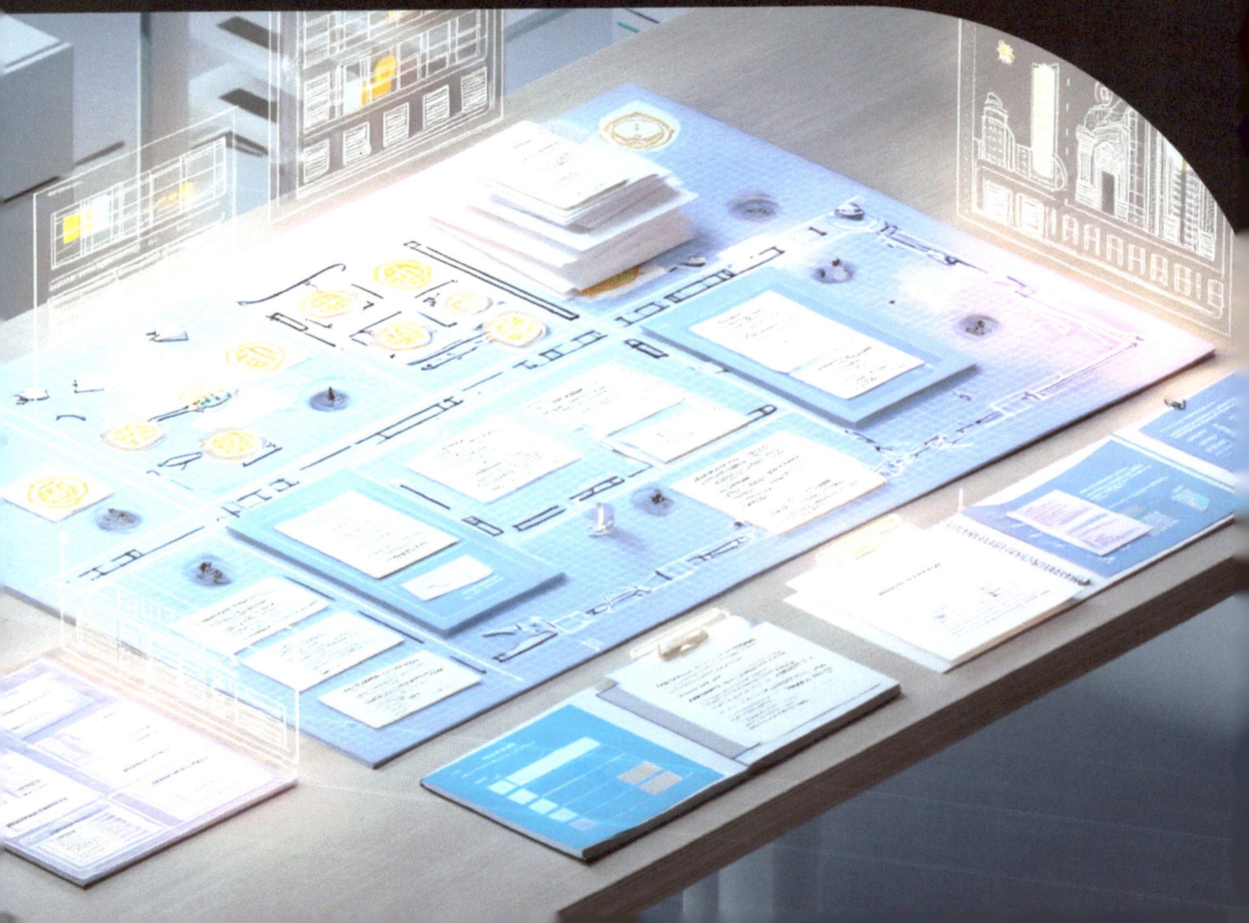

CHAPTER 19

UNDERSTANDING CALIFORNIA'S BEHAVIORAL HEALTH TRANSIFORMATION: THE BEHAVIORAL HEALTH SERVICES ACT (BHSA) AND BHCIP, BEHAVIORAL HEALTH CONTINUUM INFRASTRUCTURE PROGRAM

WHAT YOU WILL LEARN IN THIS CHAPTER:

1. What is BHSA: Behavioral Health Services Act?
2. Who BHSA helps and why?
3. BHCIP's Strategic Goals and Impacts
4. Round-by-Round Breakdown of BHCIP
5. BHCIP's Integration with California's Behavioral Health Master Plan

> "The way to get started is to quit talking and begin doing."
>
> WALT DISNEY

Vision and applied faith turn complex public programs into accessible pathways. Learn the rules, build readiness, and move when the window opens. For BHCIP, align mission, scope, and timing with program intent.

Operationalize with a readiness checklist that includes eligibility, partners, site control, program model, and capital plan. Map the scoring and prepare documents early. Coordinate with DHCS and local partners. If operating outside California, map this to your state authority and funding calendar.

THE MOMENT EVERYTHING CHANGED

It was March 2024, and I was sitting in a packed conference room in Sacramento when the results came in. Proposition 1 had passed. The Behavioral Health Infrastructure Bond Act had secured $6.38 billion in voter approval, with $4.4 billion specifically earmarked for BHCIP. After years of witnessing the crushing need for behavioral health infrastructure across California, this moment felt like a dam breaking -not of water, but of possibility.

The woman next to me, a county behavioral health director from the Central Valley, had tears in her eyes. "We've been waiting twenty years for this," she whispered. "Twenty years of patching roofs, converting closets into offices, and turning people away because we simply didn't have the space to serve them."

That moment crystallized something I'd been feeling throughout my career in behavioral health real estate: infrastructure isn't just about buildings; it's about hope made manifest in brick and mortar.

THE BEHAVIORAL HEALTH SERVICES ACT (BHSA)

WHAT IS THE BEHAVIORAL HEALTH SERVICES ACT?

The Behavioral Health Services Act replaces the Mental Health Services Act of 2004. It reforms behavioral health care funding to prioritize services for people with the most significant mental health needs while adding the treatment of substance use disorders (SUD), expanding housing interventions, and increasing the behavioral health workforce. It also enhances oversight, transparency, and accountability at the state and local levels. Additionally, the Behavioral Health Services Act creates pathways to ensure equitable access to care by advancing equity and reducing disparities for individuals with behavioral health needs. It is one part of Proposition 1. The second part of Proposition 1, the Behavioral Health Bond, authorizes $6.4 billion in bonds to finance behavioral health treatment beds, supportive housing, community sites, and funding for housing veterans with behavioral health needs.

WHAT REMAINS THE SAME FROM THE TRANSITION OF THE MENTAL HEALTH SERVICES ACT TO THE BEHAVIORAL HEALTH SERVICES ACT?

Local control to determine how funding is allocated and the community planning process for implementing services remain the same. Counties also continue to determine how services are delivered through their county system and/or through provider contractors. Counties are not required to end any of their existing contracts. Additionally, counties may choose to utilize different funding for contracts, such as Medi-Cal or other behavioral health funding sources.

The allocation methodology to distribute local funding will also stay the same. Innovation is encouraged across the Behavioral Health Services Act funding categories.

WHO WILL BE SERVED UNDER THE BEHAVIORAL HEALTH SERVICES ACT?

The Behavioral Health Services Act targets funding to provide services to eligible adults and children with or at risk of the most serious mental health conditions and SUDs, including people experiencing homelessness, at risk of incarceration, re-entering the community from a justice-involved setting, at risk of conservatorship, in foster care, and/or at risk of institutionalization.

WHY DOES THE BEHAVIORAL HEALTH SERVICES ACT EXPAND MENTAL HEALTH SERVICES ACT TO INCLUDE PEOPLE WITH SUDS?

We have come a long way in understanding SUDs and must continue to reduce the stigma associated with SUDs. The need for SUD services has increased and is often closely related to mental health conditions. Expanding eligibility to include those with SUDs provides an optional tool to address SUD service needs, based on community needs and data, such as prevalence rates. It also allows counties to use Behavioral Health Services Act funds in combination with federal funds to expand SUD service offerings.

HOW DOES THE BEHAVIORAL HEALTH SERVICES ACT SUPPORT CULTURALLY RESPONSIVE STRATEGIES AND MEET THE GOAL OF MEASURABLY REDUCING HEALTH DISPARITIES?

The Behavioral Health Services Act builds on many strategies to meet communities' needs for culturally responsive services that improve health and reduce health disparities for all, including:

- Reducing the silos for planning and service delivery.
- Requiring stratified data and strategies for reducing health disparities in planning, services, and outcomes.
- Clearly advancing community-defined practices as a key strategy for reducing health disparities and increasing diverse community representation.

HOW WILL CHILDREN AND YOUTH BENEFIT FROM THE BEHAVIORAL HEALTH SERVICES ACT?

Mental health and substance use challenges are experienced across the lifespan. The Behavioral Health Services Act strengthens tools to treat those with more serious conditions and to intervene early, meeting children, youth, and their families where they are to disrupt the trajectory toward illness and other negative outcomes. New state-administered, population-based prevention efforts will reduce the prevalence of mental health issues and SUDs and prioritize children and youth.

- High-need individuals will benefit from the emphasis on Full Service Partnerships, which provide evidence-based programs, like high-fidelity wraparound to community-defined evidence-based programs. These children and youth can benefit from a whole-person approach that is trauma-informed, age-appropriate, and in partnership with family or an individual's existing supports.
- 51 percent of early intervention funding must be directed to people 25 years of age and younger and include early childhood (0-5) mental health consultation, school-based services, and expanding early psychosis and mood disorder detection and intervention.
- Population-based programming on behavioral health and wellness to increase awareness about resources, reduce stigma, and stop behavioral health problems before they start.

WHAT ARE THE NEW RESPONSIBILITIES THE STATE IS TAKING ON WITH ITS 10 PERCENT OF ALLOCATED FUNDING?

Under the Behavioral Health Services Act there are new responsibilities for state departments:

- The California Department of Public Health (CDPH) will receive 4 percent for statewide, population-based prevention services, with 51 percent of this funding serving people 25 years of age and younger.
- The Department of Health Care Access and Information (HCAI) will receive 3 percent for sustained statewide workforce initiatives to expand a culturally competent and well-trained behavioral health workforce.

- DHCS, along with various state departments, will receive a portion of the remaining 3 percent (which was reduced from 5 percent) for oversight and monitoring, technical assistance, and administering programs. BHSOAC will direct the Innovation Partnership Fund, which sets aside $20 million annually to develop innovations with non-governmental partners.

WHAT ARE THE COUNTY FUNDING CATEGORIES UNDER THE BEHAVIORAL HEALTH SERVICES ACT?

The funding categories for county funding are as follows:

- 35 percent for Behavioral Health Services and Supports, including early intervention; outreach and engagement; workforce; education and training; capital facilities and technological needs; and innovative pilots and projects.
    - A majority (51 percent) of this amount must be used for intervention in the early signs of mental illness or SUDs.
    - A majority (51 percent) of early intervention services and supports must be for people 25 years of age and younger.

- 35 percent for Full Service Partnership programs, including comprehensive and intensive care for people at any age with the most complex needs (also known as the "whatever it takes" model).

- 30 percent for housing, including interventions for rental subsidies, operating subsidies, shared housing, family housing for eligible children and youth, and the non-federal share of certain transitional rent.
    - Half of this amount (50 percent) is prioritized for housing interventions for the chronically homeless.
    - Up to 25 percent may be used for capital development.

- Provides counties with flexibility within the above funding areas by allowing each county to move up to 7 percent from one category to another, for a maximum of 14 percent more added into any one category, to allow counties to address their different local needs and priorities – based on data and community input.

COUNTIES ARE VERY DIFFERENT, ESPECIALLY SMALL COUNTIES. ARE THERE OTHER FLEXIBILITIES OR EXEMPTIONS?

Yes, counties have unique strengths and challenges, especially small counties with a population of 200,000 or less. With input from counties, DHCS will develop criteria and create an approval process for small county exemptions. Two key examples include:

- An exemption from dedicating 30 percent of local funds for housing interventions in the 2026-29 planning cycle and ongoing.
- An exemption from providing certain treatment models at fidelity that small counties may not have the capacity or scale to provide.

HOW DOES THE BEHAVIORAL HEALTH SERVICES ACT IMPROVE OVERSIGHT, ACCOUNTABILITY, AND TRANSPARENCY TO THE PUBLIC?

There are two significant updates that help accomplish these goals.

- County Integrated Plan for Behavioral Health Services and Outcomes: These three-year planning documents, the first of which a draft is due March 31, 2026, and the final due June 30, 2026, will provide a more comprehensive and transparent picture of all public local, state, and federal behavioral health funding, including Behavioral Health Services Act, Realignment, federal Substance Abuse and Mental Health Services Administration and Projects for Assistance in Transition from Homelessness (PATH) grants, opioid settlement funds, and Medi-Cal. The plans will provide a budget of planned expenditures, reserves, and adjustments, align with state and local goals and outcome measures, and outline workforce strategies. Plans must be informed by local stakeholder input, including additional voices on the local behavioral health advisory boards.

- County Behavioral Health Outcomes, Accountability, and Transparency Report: Counties will be required to report annually on expenditures of all local, state, and federal behavioral health funding (e.g., Behavioral Health Services Act, Realignment funding, federal Substance Abuse and Mental Health Services Administration and PATH grants, opioid settlement funds, and Medi-Cal), unspent dollars, service utilization data and outcomes with a health equity lens, workforce metrics, and other information. DHCS is authorized to impose corrective action plans on counties failing to meet certain requirements.

Performance outcomes will be developed by DHCS in consultation with counties and stakeholders. An additional 2 percent and up to 4 percent for small counties of local Behavioral Health Services Act revenue may be used to improve planning, quality, outcomes, data reporting, and subcontractor oversight for all county behavioral health funding, on top of the existing 5 percent county planning allotment. Counties can also use funds to support training and technical assistance to ensure stakeholders have enough information and data to participate in the development of integrated plans and annual updates.

WHERE SHOULD I START IF I'M SEEKING MENTAL HEALTH AND/OR SUD TREATMENT?

If you're seeking services for mental health and SUD services, please visit the DHCS website for information on available resources and treatment options. The 988 Suicide and Crisis Lifeline is available 24 hours a day, seven days a week, 365 days a year. You may also connect with CalHOPEby live chat, call (833) 317-HOPE (4673), or text. Additionally, a groundbreaking new program provides free, safe, and confidential mental health support for young people and families across the state with two easy-to-use mobile apps: BrightLife Kids and Soluna.

Further, Shatterproof Treatment Atlas, an addiction treatment locator, assessment, and standards platform, can connect individuals to appropriate evidence-based addiction treatment. To empower individuals and change attitudes about SUDs, DHCS launched Unshame California, a science-driven and content-based campaign that promotes anti-stigma messaging through stories of Californians impacted by SUDs. Both Treatment Atlas and Unshame California align with ongoing statewide initiatives to reduce substance use overdoses, support recovery efforts, and educate the public.

I. Overview of the Behavioral Health Continuum Infrastructure Program (BHCIP)

The Behavioral Health Continuum Infrastructure Program (BHCIP) emerged from a perfect storm of necessity, political will, and strategic vision. Established by Assembly Bill 133 and Senate Bill 129 in 2021 and dramatically expanded by the passage of Proposition 1 in 2024, BHCIP represents the largest behavioral health infrastructure initiative in California's history. Administered by the Department of Health Care Services (DHCS) with technical assistance from Advocates for Human Potential (AHP), the program provides billions of dollars to construct and renovate facilities across the care continuum.

II. BHCIP's Strategic Goals and Impacts

BHCIP aims to create modern, community-based behavioral health facilities, prioritizing the state's most vulnerable populations, including justice-involved individuals, foster youth, and those experiencing homelessness. The program's goal is to build a flexible continuum of care, from crisis stabilization to residential treatment, that reduces fragmentation and addresses geographic disparities in service availability.

III. Round-by-Round Breakdown of BHCIP

Understanding BHCIP requires appreciating how each funding round addresses specific needs:

- BHCIP Bond Round 1 (Launch Ready) - $3.3 Billion: This unprecedented investment targets projects that can break ground immediately, requiring demonstration of site control, completed environmental review, and secured local approvals. ~ 124 Awards delivered May 6, 2025.

· BHCIP Bond Round 2 (Unmet Needs) - $800+ Million: Specifically targeting rural and underserved areas, Round 2 addresses geographic disparities in behavioral health infrastructure. The application period opened in June 2025 with an October 2025 deadline.

· BHCIP Rounds 3-5 - $2.2 Billion: These earlier rounds focused on planning grants, crisis and continuum infrastructure, and programs for individuals with co-occurring developmental disabilities, laying the groundwork for the larger bond-funded initiatives. ~133 Awards delivered June 2022 - March 2024

IV. Role of DHCS and AHP in Program Implementation

DHCS serves as the primary program administrator, providing oversight and funding, while AHP provides crucial technical assistance, application review, and peer learning facilitation. The mandatory Pre-Application Consultation (PAC) process, managed by AHP, ensures that projects are properly scoped and aligned with community needs before formal submission.

V. BHCIP Program Milestones and Outcomes

The BHCIP initiative is on track to create thousands of new residential beds and outpatient facility spaces across California. The initial rounds have already funded over 250 projects, representing a significant expansion of the state's capacity to deliver care. Success is measured not just in square footage but in the ability of these new facilities to integrate with broader state policies and improve client outcomes.

VI. The Grant Lifecycle: From Application to Activation

The BHCIP grant lifecycle is a multi-stage process:

Pre-Award:

Applicants conduct feasibility studies, secure site control, and develop a clear project vision.

Application:

Following a mandatory PAC, applicants submit detailed proposals through AHP's portal.

Award & Contracting:

Successful grantees enter into a formal agreement with the state, locking in a milestone-based funding schedule.

Post-Award Execution:

Grantees proceed with construction under strict monitoring, providing regular progress reports to DHCS.

VII. Lessons Learned from BHCIP Rounds

Early rounds have highlighted several key success factors, including the importance of strong Owners' Advisors, early site control, and robust stakeholder alignment. Common pitfalls include underestimating project costs and, most critically, failing to address licensing requirements early in the process -a topic covered in detail in Chapter 20 .

VIII. BHCIP's Integration with California's Behavioral Health Master Plan

BHCIP's true power emerges through its integration with California's broader behavioral health transformation initiatives, including CalAIM (California Advancing and Innovating Medi-Cal) and the CARE (Community Assistance, Recovery & Empowerment) Court. BHCIP provides the physical infrastructure necessary for these new service delivery models to succeed, creating a tangible foundation for policy innovation. Furthermore, the statutory CEQA exemptions provided under WIC §5960.3 have been a game-changer, dramatically accelerating project timelines.

IX. Strategic Opportunities Ahead

The passage of Proposition 1 and the launch of BHCIP Round 2 for "Unmet Needs" signal a long-term commitment to rebuilding California's behavioral health infrastructure. Future opportunities lie in leveraging the lessons from BHCIP to inform federal policy, scale successful facility models, and foster innovative public-private partnerships that ensure operational sustainability long after construction is complete.

X. Case Studies of Impact

· Alameda Health System: A $77+ million award is supporting a regional-scale integration, expanding psychiatric emergency services and creating new residential and outpatient capacity. The project exemplifies how BHCIP can transform an entire county's service delivery system.

· Napa County: A $3.3 million Crisis Stabilization Unit illustrates how BHCIP addresses the unique challenges of rural communities, with a flexible design that allows the facility to serve multiple functions.

· BACS (Alameda County): A $32 million award for a state-of-the-art behavioral health center showcases innovation in community-based care, incorporating trauma-informed design and extensive technology integration.

As California moves forward, BHCIP provides more than just funding; it offers a blueprint for how to build a more equitable, accessible, and compassionate system of care -one facility at a time.

Chapter 20

LICENSING in Behavioral Health Real Estate

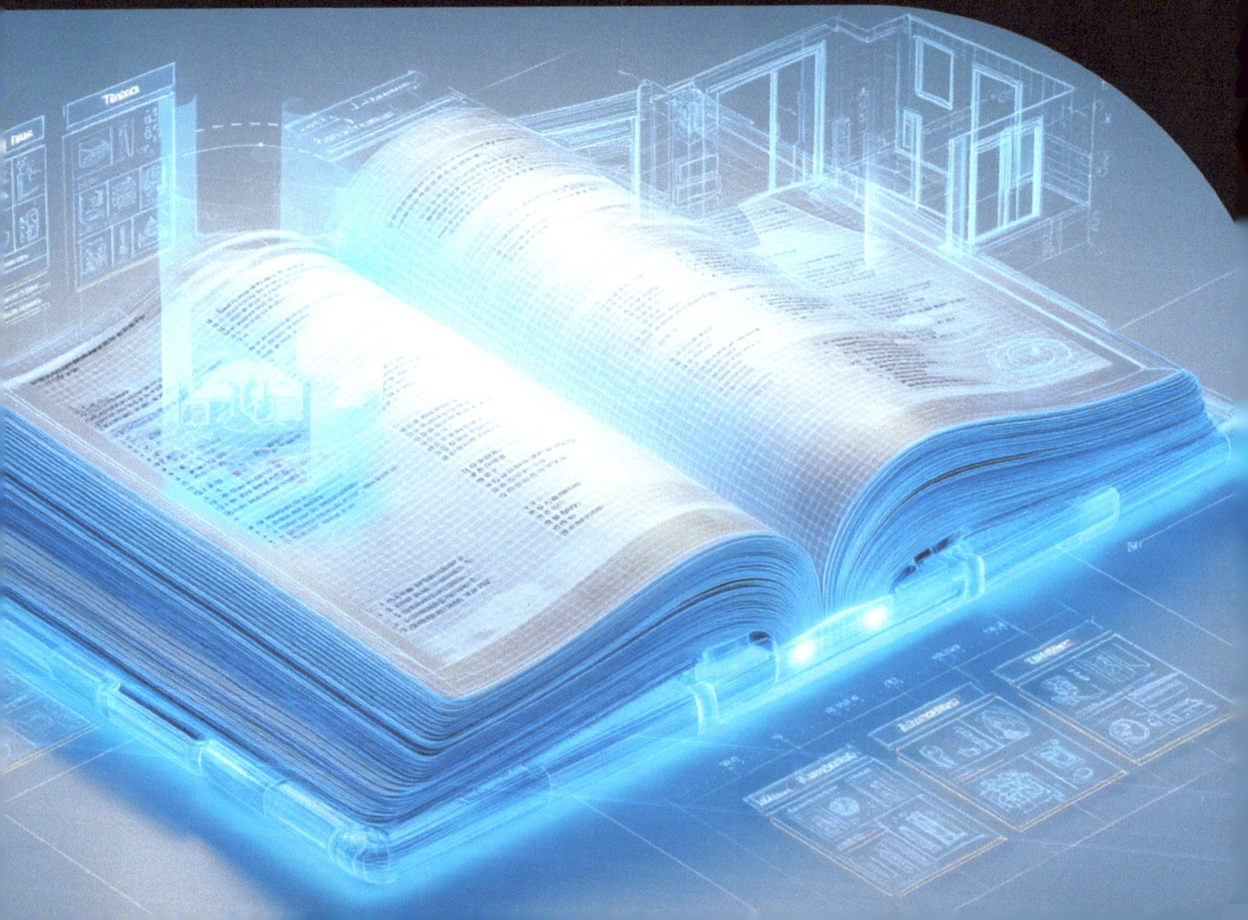

CHAPTER 20
LICENSING IN BEHAVIORAL HEALTH REAL ESTATE

WHAT YOU WILL LEARN IN THIS CHAPTER:

- Licensing Is Central to Real Estate Strategy
- Facility Types and Their Licensing Implications
- The Licensing Application Process: A Step-by-Step Guide
- Building Legally Operable, Fundable, and Compliant Facilities in California

"The time to repair the roof is when the sun is shining."

JOHN F. KENNEDY

CHAPTER OVERVIEW

Licensing is one of the most consequential components in behavioral health facility development. No matter how visionary the project, if it fails to align with California licensing regulations, it cannot open, operate, or bill for services. This chapter provides a practical, step-by-step guide for navigating the licensing landscape across DHCS, CDSS, and HCAI, especially when aligning with large-scale funding initiatives like BHCIP. It explores license types, application pathways, and how facility design, funding, and licensability must be harmonized for a project to succeed.

Organized knowledge and persistence carry licensing across the finish line. Demonstrate readiness with calm, complete evidence. In behavioral health, licensing is a process you lead with checklists, training, and respectful agency coordination.

Turn mindset into a Licensing Book that mirrors requirements and shows compliance clearly. Prepare staff, policies, and physical plant in sequence. Track corrective actions to closure. If operating outside California, map this to your state authority and funding calendar.

I. WHY LICENSING IS CENTRAL TO REAL ESTATE STRATEGY

In behavioral health development, a license is more than a piece of paper; it is the legal key that unlocks a facility's ability to operate. It is the "go/no-go" threshold that separates a completed building from a functioning center for care. While zoning exemptions like those under Welfare and Institutions Code § 5960.3 can streamline local planning approvals, they do not eliminate the rigorous state-level licensing obligations. This is especially true for projects seeking funding through major state initiatives like BHCIP, which is explored in depth in Chapter 19 . The Owner's Advisor plays a critical role in ensuring this licensability from day one, aligning architectural plans, clinical programs, and financial models with the specific requirements of the target license.

II. MAJOR STATE LICENSING AGENCIES IN CALIFORNIA

Navigating California's regulatory environment requires understanding the roles of three key agencies:

- **DHCS** (Department of Health Care Services): This agency oversees higher-acuity clinical programs that are more medical in nature. These include Adult Residential Treatment Facilities (ARTF), Crisis Residential

Treatment Programs (CRT), Mental Health Rehabilitation Centers (MHRC), Psychiatric Health Facilities (PHF), and most residential substance use disorder (SUD) programs.

- **CDSS/CCL** (Department of Social Services, Community Care Licensing Division):CDSS generally oversees lower-acuity, non-medical residential care programs. These include Adult Residential Facilities (ARFs), Residential Care Facilities for the Elderly (RCFEs), and Short-Term Residential Therapeutic Programs (STRTPs) for youth.
- **HCAI** (Department of Health Care Access and Information): Formerly OSHPD, HCAI is not a primary program licensor but is a critical partner. HCAI reviews and approves the physical plant (the building itself) for certain licensed facilities, like PHFs, ensuring compliance with hospital-level seismic safety and construction standards.

III. FACILITY TYPES AND THEIR LICENSING IMPLICATIONS

The choice of license type is a strategic decision that dictates everything from staffing ratios and room configurations to reimbursement rates. The program model must drive the real estate, not the other way around.

IV. LICENSING AND THE BHCIP PERFORMANCE LIFECYCLE

For projects funded by BHCIP, licensing alignment is a contractual obligation. The license you apply for must match the program model described in your BHCIP funding award. A misalignment can lead to severe consequences, including the loss of funding, denial of a Certificate of Occupancy, or major construction delays. The Owner's Advisor is responsible for ensuring this alignment is established in pre-construction, harmonizing the project scope, the use of funds, the facility classification, and the licensing submission timeline.

V. THE LICENSING APPLICATION PROCESS: A STEP-BY-STEP GUIDE

The licensing process is methodical and can typically take between 90 and 150 days, assuming no major issues arise.

Feasibility and Classification Analysis:

Confirm your program's intent and match it to a specific license type. This will inform the building layout, including bedroom counts, security zones, and staffing areas.

Pre-Application:

Engage with DHCS or CDSS early. These informal consultations provide invaluable feedback on your plans before you make costly mistakes.

Plan Review:

For higher-acuity facilities, HCAI will conduct a detailed review of your architectural and engineering plans to ensure compliance with physical plant requirements.

Formal Application:

Submit a detailed Program Narrative and a Policy & Procedure Manual that describes exactly how your facility will operate.

Pre-Licensing Inspection:

Once your application is accepted, a state licensing analyst will conduct an on-site inspection to ensure the physical facility matches your plans and meets all life-safety codes.

Final Licensing Approval:

Upon a successful inspection, the state will issue the license, allowing you to officially open and begin providing services.

VI. LICENSING CONSIDERATIONS DURING DESIGN AND CONSTRUCTION

Licensing requirements must be integrated into the design from the very beginning. Common conflicts often arise between the desire for open, therapeutic environments and the need for security and safety. For example, an open floor plan might be excellent for community building, but it can create challenges for staff-to-patient sightlines and security. An experienced architect and owner's advisor can help navigate these trade-offs, ensuring the final design is both healing and compliant.

VII. THE FINANCIAL IMPLICATIONS OF LICENSING

The license type directly impacts a facility's financial model. It determines Medi-Cal reimbursement rates, eligibility for certain grants, and qualified uses of capital funding. For most providers, licensability is the absolute precondition for financial sustainability. Without the correct license, you cannot bill for services, certify your bed count, or contract with private payers.

VIII. FUTURE DIRECTIONS IN CALIFORNIA LICENSING POLICY

The regulatory landscape is always evolving. Between 2025 and 2027, both DHCS and HCAI are working toward streamlining their processes through digital application systems. There is also a growing emphasis in licensing regulations on creating trauma-informed care environments. We are also seeing the emergence of new licensing pathways for innovative models like "Behavioral Health Urgent Care" (BHUC), transitional housing with co-located services, and peer-run respite centers. Staying ahead of these trends is critical for future-proofing your facility.

CONCLUSION: LICENSING AS THE FOUNDATION OF TRUST

In behavioral health real estate, a license is more than a permit to operate. It is a promise to the community, to regulators, and to the vulnerable individuals you serve. It is a declaration that your facility is safe, your program is sound, and your team is ready to provide compassionate, high-quality care. Navigating this complex process requires expertise, foresight, and a relentless commitment to getting the details right. With a skilled Owner's Advisor to guide the way, you can build facilities that are not only compliant and fundable, but are true sanctuaries for healing.

Chapter 21

The Call to **ACTION** for Leaders and Communities

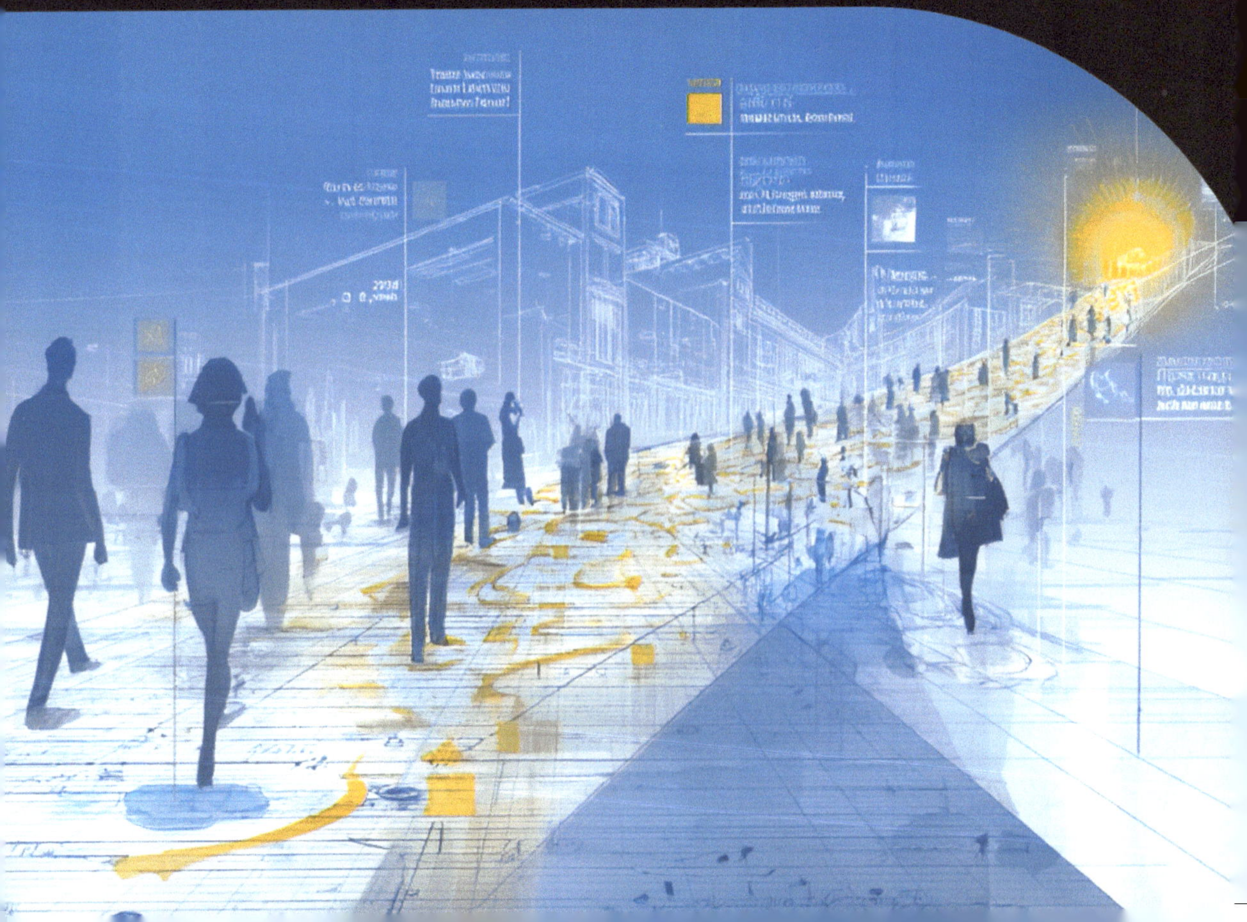

CHAPTER 21
CALL TO ACTION FOR BEHAVIORAL HEALTH INFRASTRUCTURE

WHAT YOU WILL LEARN:

- The Growing Urgency for Behavioral Health Infrastructure
- The Imperative of Subject Matter Expertise
- The Call to Action: Building a New Era of Care

1. BUILDING A NEW ERA OF CARE

> "The future belongs to those who believe in the beauty of their dreams."
>
> ELEANOR ROOSEVELT

The vision for the future of behavioral health infrastructure is one of integration, not isolation. For too long, we have built facilities that stand apart from the community, reinforcing stigma and creating barriers to care. The next era will be defined by smaller, more flexible facilities that are woven into the fabric of our neighborhoods. Imagine a community wellness hub on a busy corner, co-locating mental health services with primary care, a healthy café, and even affordable housing upstairs. Picture mobile crisis teams dispatched from decentralized hubs, meeting people where they are, rather than forcing them into an intimidating emergency room.

This future requires a new kind of developer and a new kind of leader. It requires experts who can navigate the complexities of mixed-use financing, who can build partnerships between healthcare systems and housing authorities, and who can design spaces that are technologically enabled for telehealth and data-driven care. My role as an Owner's Advisor is to be a catalyst for this change: to be the integrator who brings these diverse partners to the table and helps them build the compassionate, accessible, and integrated infrastructure that our future demands.

2. THE URGENCY FOR EXPERTISE

> "The expert in anything was once a beginner."
>
> HELEN HAYES

I was once brought into a project that was on the brink of failure. It was a well-intentioned effort to build a residential treatment center, led by a passionate group with no prior development experience. They had bought the wrong property, hired the wrong architect, and completely misunderstood the state's licensing requirements. Their good intentions had led them to the edge of a financial and regulatory cliff. We were able to salvage the project, but it cost them dearly in time, money, and stress.

That experience solidified my belief that the growing mental health crisis demands more than just passion; it demands a higher standard of professional expertise. We cannot afford to learn on the job when people's lives are at stake. My commitment, and the purpose of this book, is to help build that expertise. It is to share the lessons learned from both successes and failures, to elevate the standards of our field, and to mentor the next generation of developers, builders, and advisors. The urgency of this moment requires us to be not just passionate but professional; not just well-meaning but well-informed. Our communities deserve nothing less.

3. A MOMENT OF OPPORTUNITY

We are in a time of great change for behavioral health. Awareness about mental health is rising, but many communities still don't have the facilities to meet the need. That gap is growing, and so is the urgency to act.

Every year, millions of people across the country struggle with mental health conditions and substance use. Families are impacted, hospitals are overcrowded, and people are waiting too long to get help. It doesn't have to be this way. Behavioral health facilities aren't just buildings; they are places of hope and healing. They shape how care is delivered, how people feel, and how recovery begins.

4. "WHY EXPERTISE MATTERS"

Building a behavioral health facility takes more than good intentions. It takes experience and knowledge across many areas: healthcare, design, funding, policy, and local relationships. The most successful projects are led by teams that understand:

- How to design safe, calming spaces
- How to work through city and state approvals
- How to find and manage complex funding sources
- How to partner with the community

A Real-World Example

In South Los Angeles, one project faced major roadblocks with local resistance, complicated zoning, and funding issues. But an experienced team stepped in and turned things around. They held open conversations with neighbors and gained support. They used smart strategies to navigate zoning approvals. They created a funding plan that combined federal, state, and private dollars. Now, that facility helps thousands of people each year. It shows what's possible when a skilled team is aligned with a clear purpose.

WHAT MAKES A PROJECT WORK

Every successful behavioral health facility rests on a few essential principles.

1. Plan Across Disciplines

- Use **real data** to define needs.
- Develop a **long-term budget** covering both construction and operations.
- Prepare early for **licensing and compliance** requirements.

2. Involve the Community

- **Listen first**: communities are partners, not just stakeholders.
- Be **open and transparent** from the outset.
- Collaborate with **local leaders** who already have community trust.

3. Design for Healing & Flexibility

- Create environments that are **safe, open, and calming**.
- Ensure designs can **adapt as care models evolve**.
- Integrate **sustainability and energy efficiency** from day one.

4. Moving Forward Together

No single group can solve the behavioral health crisis. Progress requires governments, healthcare leaders, developers, and communities working as one.

A. Align Funding & Policy

- Strengthen programs like **Medi-Cal** and **CalAIM**.
- **Simplify approval processes** for facilities.
- Provide **incentives** for developers who build healing spaces.

B. Stay Open to Innovation

- Plan facilities with **future care models** in mind: telehealth, mobile crisis teams, digital tools.
- Use **data and technology** to improve both care delivery and operations.

Summary: Projects work best when they are **planned holistically, rooted in community, designed for healing, and supported by aligned policy and innovation.**

CONCLUSION: THE WELLSPRING PROMISE

This book is a guide, and it is also an invitation. Building behavioral health infrastructure is not only technical work. It is meaningful work that improves the lives of patients, families, and entire communities.

Every project you advance is a public statement that healing is possible and that access to care is a right. Each site plan, permit, and punch list moves that promise from idea to reality.

If you are reading this, you have a role. Builder, policymaker, provider, investor, advocate, neighbor. What you do next matters.

Move forward with care, courage, and collaboration. Hold the mission steady. Welcome community voices. Design for dignity. Deliver with discipline. Measure what matters, learn, and keep improving.

Let us build places that heal.

Let us build the capacity our communities deserve.

Let us build what the future needs.

ABOUT THE AUTHOR, BRIAN JONES

"You must be the change you wish to see in the world"

MAHATMA GANDHI

This book is not the story of one person -it's a reflection of many. It was written in the spirit of collaboration, with the belief that real change in behavioral health care comes from communities coming together with purpose, vision, and care.

At the heart of this work is Brian Jones, a dedicated member of a growing circle of behavioral health professionals, advocates, and healers who believe in building spaces that foster recovery and hope. With over two decades of experience in real estate development, behavioral health consulting, and systems planning, Brian's journey has always been grounded in service -to people, to purpose, and to possibility.

But the work featured in these pages is not his alone. It has been shaped by the wisdom of clinicians, the courage of community leaders, the insight of architects and planners, and the quiet determination of individuals who know that better is possible. It is the shared effort of a few committed people working toward something larger than themselves.

A LIFE IN COLLABORATION

Brian's professional path has taken him through many sectors -from housing and healthcare to policy and construction. As the founder of BHSME, LLC, he has supported the development of behavioral health facilities across California and beyond, helping turn visions into reality. His work spans concept planning, project management, strategic funding, stakeholder engagement, and real estate development, always with the goal of creating environments that support healing and belonging.

He lives on a small organic farm in San Diego with his fiancé, their dog, cat, bees, fruit trees, and gardens - a life that mirrors the values he brings to his work: sustainability, connection, and care.

His background includes studies in psychology, religion, personality theory, and sustainable real estate. He holds degrees from Stanford University and advanced training in psychology and real estate development, blending the academic with the practical in his approach to healing-centered infrastructure.

A PRACTICE OF SHARED VISION

While Brian has led large-scale development projects and advised state agencies and nonprofit leaders, what matters most to him is teamwork. The best outcomes, he believes, are always the result of many people working together -listening, adapting, and building in response to real community needs.

At BHSME, that belief is embedded in everything they do. From early-stage planning to final construction, projects are guided by the wisdom of teams who value equity, sustainability, trauma-informed design, and deep respect for the lived experience of those they serve.

A BROADER MISSION

Behavioral health care is not just a sector -it's a movement. A movement toward more inclusive, accessible, and compassionate systems of care. Brian's work supports this mission by helping communities design spaces that feel safe, welcoming, and empowering.

He believes in:

Co-creation with community voices

Healing-centered design that meets people where they are

Innovative infrastructure that can adapt to the changing needs of care

His vision is simple: build places that help people get better, and support the teams that make that healing possible.

FINAL THOUGHTS

This book is a reflection of what's possible when people come together to solve hard problems with heart, knowledge, and humility. It is not a blueprint from above -it's a shared resource from the field. A tool for those who believe that the future of behavioral health must be built, not just hoped for.

Brian offers this work in gratitude -to everyone working quietly and persistently to bring healing into the world. To the frontline caregivers, the project managers, the advocates, and the public servants. To the communities that open their doors and their minds to new possibilities.

If you find hope, ideas, or practical guidance in these pages, know that you are already part of this movement. Together, we are building something that matters.

With appreciation and solidarity,

Brian Jones Founder, BHSME, LLC
www.bhsme.org brian@bhsme.org

GLOSSARY OF REAL ESTATE DEVELOPMENT TERMS

A working glossary for “The Wellspring”

GLOSSARY OF REAL ESTATE DEVELOPMENT TERMS

A

- **ADA (Americans with Disabilities Act):** Federal accessibility standards that shape design and operations.
- **AHJ (Authority Having Jurisdiction):** The agency or official that interprets and enforces codes and approvals.
- **ALTA/NSPS Land Title Survey:** Detailed survey showing boundaries, easements, encroachments, setbacks, and access, coordinated with the title report.
- **Appraisal:** Independent opinion of property value used for financing and acquisitions.
- **Architectural Test Fit:** Early space planning study to confirm that the program fits a site or existing building.
- **As-Built Drawings:** Record drawings that document final constructed conditions.
- **Absorption:** Rate at which space is leased or units are occupied in the market.

B

- **Basis of Design (BOD):** Written and diagrammatic narrative defining the design intent and system criteria.
- **BIM (Building Information Modeling):** 3D model used for coordination, clash detection, quantities, and life cycle tracking.
- **Bond:** Debt instrument used to finance projects; surety bonds may guarantee performance or payment.
- **Brownfield:** Property complicated by real or perceived environmental contamination.
- **Builder’s Risk Insurance:** Property coverage for buildings under construction.
- **Building Permit:** Official authorization to construct per approved plans.

C

- **C of O or CO (Certificate of Occupancy):** Jurisdictional sign-off allowing legal occupancy.

- **CC&R (Covenants, Conditions, and Restrictions):** Recorded limitations that affect property use.
- **CEQA (California Environmental Quality Act):** State environmental review for discretionary approvals.
- **Change Order:** Written modification to scope, price, or schedule after contract execution.
- **Conditional Use Permit (CUP):** Discretionary approval for uses not permitted by right.
- **Constructability Review:** Multidisciplinary review to identify design conflicts before bidding.
- **Construction Documents (CDs):** Drawings and specifications used for permitting, bidding, and construction.
- **Contingency:** Budget or schedule reserve for unknowns and risk.
- **Cost of Work:** Direct construction costs excluding fee, general conditions, and bonds.
- **Critical Path Method (CPM):** Schedule technique that identifies activities controlling project duration.
- **Capital Stack:** Combination of grants, tax credits, debt, and equity used to finance a project.

D

- **Davis-Bacon:** Federal prevailing wage requirements on applicable projects.
- **Demolition:** Deconstruction of existing improvements before renovation or new work.
- **Design-Bid-Build (DBB):** Traditional delivery with separate design and construction contracts.
- **Design-Build (DB):** Single contract for design and construction.
- **Developer Fee:** Compensation to the developer for organizing and delivering the project.
- **Developer Overhead:** General business expenses not tied to a specific project task.
- **Development Planning:** Ongoing refinement of scope, schedule, and budget through design phases.
- **DIR Registration:** Required California contractor registration for public works with prevailing wage.
- **Draw Request:** Formal request to a lender or funder for disbursement of construction funds.
- **Due Diligence:** Comprehensive investigations to confirm feasibility and risk.

E

- **Easement:** Legal right for another party to use a portion of property for access or utilities.
- **Earned Value Management (EVM):** Method to track schedule and budget performance.
- **EIR (Environmental Impact Report):** CEQA document analyzing significant impacts and mitigations.
- **Entitlements:** Discretionary approvals such as CUPs, variances, and map approvals.

- **Environmental Site Assessment Phase I:** Desktop review and site reconnaissance to identify potential contamination.
- **Environmental Site Assessment Phase II:** Sampling and lab analysis when Phase I finds recognized environmental concerns.
- **Equity:** Ownership capital invested in a project.
- **Escrow:** Neutral third party that manages documents and funds during transactions.

F

- **FAR (Floor Area Ratio):** Ratio of building floor area to site area that controls density.
- **Feasibility Study:** Market, cost, and regulatory analysis to test viability.
- **FF&E (Furniture, Fixtures, and Equipment):** Movable items required for operations near project closeout.
- **Force Majeure:** Events beyond control that may excuse delays or nonperformance.
- **Funding Agreement:** Contract detailing terms, conditions, and reporting for project funding.

G

- **Gantt Chart:** Bar chart showing schedule activities and durations.
- **General Conditions or Requirements:** Indirect job costs such as supervision, temporary utilities, insurance, and administration.
- **General Contractor (GC):** Entity responsible for means and methods, safety, and subcontract management.
- **Geotechnical Report:** Soil borings and analysis that inform foundations, grading, and pavement.
- **GMP (Guaranteed Maximum Price):** Contract sum cap with defined allowances, contingencies, and savings provisions.
- **Greenfield:** Undeveloped site with no prior construction.
- **Ground-Up Construction:** New building on previously undeveloped land.

H

- **HCAI (California Department of Health Care Access and Information):** State oversight for certain health facilities and construction.
- **Hard Bid:** Competitive bidding based on complete documents and low price selection.
- **Hard Costs:** Direct construction costs such as grading, concrete, structure, MEP, and landscaping.
- **HUD (U.S. Department of Housing and Urban Development):** Federal housing programs and financing.

I

- **ICRA (Infection Control Risk Assessment):** Plan to control infection risk during construction in healthcare settings.
- **Impact Fees:** One-time fees to mitigate project impacts on public infrastructure.
- **Indemnity:** Contract obligation to protect another party against specified claims or losses.
- **Insurance Requirements:** Contract provisions for liability, builder's risk, workers' compensation, and professional liability.
- **Intensive Outpatient Treatment (IOT):** Nonresidential program providing at least nine hours of treatment per week.
- **IOR (Inspector of Record):** HCAI-approved inspector overseeing code and plan compliance.

J

- **Joint Venture (JV):** Partnership between entities to share risk, cost, and returns.
- **Jurisdiction:** Government body with authority over land use, building, or health approvals.

L

- **Land Costs or Value:** Purchase price or appraised value used in underwriting.
- **Lease Types:** Gross, modified gross, and triple-net structures that define expense responsibilities.
- **Lender's PCA (Property Condition Assessment):** Third-party building evaluation for lenders.
- **Letter of Intent (LOI):** Nonbinding agreement that outlines proposed terms before a definitive contract.
- **Level of Care Designation:** Regulatory approval defining services a facility may provide.
- **Lien Waiver:** Document from contractors or suppliers waiving lien rights upon payment.
- **Liquidated Damages:** Pre-agreed daily amount owed for late completion.
- **Loan-to-Value (LTV):** Loan amount divided by appraised value.

M

- **Master Plan:** Long-range plan for phasing, circulation, utilities, and growth.
- **Mechanic's Lien:** Security interest in property for unpaid labor or materials.
- **MEP (Mechanical, Electrical, Plumbing):** Engineering disciplines for building systems.
- **Mitigated Negative Declaration (MND):** CEQA finding that impacts are reduced to less than significant.

- **Memorandum of Understanding (MOU):** Nonbinding document outlining roles and responsibilities.
- **MMRP (Mitigation Monitoring and Reporting Program):** CEQA compliance plan for adopted mitigations.

N

- **NEPA (National Environmental Policy Act):** Federal environmental review for projects with federal nexus.
- **Net Operating Income (NOI):** Income after operating expenses and before debt service.
- **NIMBY:** Local opposition to development near existing neighborhoods.
- **Notice to Proceed (NTP):** Owner's authorization for the contractor to start work.

O

- **OAC Meeting (Owner-Architect-Contractor):** Regular coordination meeting for design and construction issues.
- **OCIP or CCIP:** Owner-controlled or contractor-controlled wrap-up insurance covering multiple parties.
- **O&M (Operations and Maintenance):** Procedures, manuals, and staffing for ongoing operation.
- **Owner's Contingency:** Reserve controlled by the owner for scope or pricing unknowns.
- **Owner's Representative or Advisor:** Professional acting on the owner's behalf for strategy, risk, and coordination.

P

- **Pay Application or Pay App:** Contractor's monthly request for payment based on work completed.
- **Permit Fees:** Charges for plan review and permit issuance based on scope and valuation.
- **Phasing Plan:** Sequenced approach to design, construction, and activation.
- **Physical Needs Assessment (PNA):** Building condition survey with repair scope and costs.
- **Predevelopment:** Early work such as due diligence, schematics, budgets, and permitting strategy.
- **Preliminary Budget:** Early cost model based on square-foot factors and assumptions.
- **Prevailing Wages:** Government-set wage and fringe rates for public works.
- **Procurement Methods:** RFQ, RFP, negotiated selection, or best-value selection.
- **Program or Programming:** Quantification of space, adjacencies, and performance requirements.
- **Pro Forma:** Financial projection of revenues, expenses, capital costs, and returns.

- **Project Inspection Costs:** Fees for jurisdictional, funder, and specialty inspections.
- **Punch List:** List of incomplete or deficient items to finish before final completion.

Q

- **QA/QC (Quality Assurance and Quality Control):** Systems and reviews that verify compliance with design and standards.
- **QAP (Qualified Allocation Plan):** State criteria for allocating Low-Income Housing Tax Credits.

R

- **Record Drawings:** Marked-up plans that capture field changes for closeout.
- **Reasonable Costs:** Actual costs that do not exceed market rates for comparable services.
- **Request for Information (RFI):** Formal question to clarify documents during bidding or construction.
- **Request for Proposals (RFP):** Solicitation outlining scope and evaluation for services.
- **Request for Qualifications (RFQ):** Solicitation focusing on experience and capability.
- **Right of Way (ROW):** Land reserved for public access or utilities.

S

- **Schematic Design (SD):** Concept phase producing plans, key elevations, outline specs, and preliminary budgets.
- **Schedule of Values (SOV):** Line-item breakdown of contract value used for payment approvals.
- **Scope Creep:** Uncontrolled expansion of work outside approved scope.
- **Soft Costs:** Nonconstruction costs such as design, permitting, testing, legal, and financing.
- **Stormwater Pollution Prevention Plan (SWPPP):** Required plan for erosion and sediment control.
- **Submittals:** Product data, samples, and shop drawings for design compliance review.
- **Substantial Completion:** Stage when work is sufficiently complete for intended use, often tied to TCO.
- **Survey:** Field measurement of property boundaries and features.

T

- **Takeoff:** Quantity measurement for estimating materials and labor.
- **Tax Credits:** Incentives such as LIHTC and NMTC used in capital stacks.

- **Temporary Certificate of Occupancy (TCO):** Conditional approval for limited occupancy before final CO.
- **Title 24:** California energy code and building standards.
- **Title Report (Preliminary):** Ownership, liens, easements, and encumbrances affecting title.
- **Traffic Impact Analysis (TIA):** Study of project traffic effects and required mitigations.

U

- **Underwriting:** Lender or investor analysis of risks, returns, and assumptions.
- **Use Permit:** Approval for specific land uses that are not permitted by right.
- **Utility Will-Serve Letter:** Utility confirmation of capacity and connection conditions.

V

- **Value Engineering (VE):** Structured review to achieve required performance at the lowest life-cycle cost.
- **Variance:** Approval to deviate from a specific zoning standard.

W

- **Warranty:** Contractor or manufacturer obligation to repair or replace defective work.
- **Work Letter:** Lease exhibit defining tenant improvements, allowances, and delivery conditions.
- **Wrap-Up Insurance:** Consolidated insurance program covering multiple parties on a project.

Z

- **Zoning Map Amendment:** Legislative change to a property's zoning designation.
- **Zoning Ordinance:** Local code governing land use, density, height, parking, and setbacks.

RESOURCES FOR BEHAVIORAL HEALTH REAL ESTATE DEVELOPMENT SUPPORT IN CALIFORNIA

Quick directory: Each entry lists a website and phone number.

American Planning Association (APA), California Chapter
Website: apacalifornia.org
Phone: (916) 448-6859

Associated Builders and Contractors (ABC)
Website: abc.org
Phone: (703) 812-2000

Behavioral Health Subject Matter Experts (BHSME)
Website: bhsme.org
Phone: (415) 269-5357

California Association of Local Agency Formation Commissions (CALAFCO)
Website: calafco.org
Phone: (916) 442-6536

California Association for Local Economic Development (CALED)
Website: caled.org
Phone: (916) 448-8252

California Association of Nonprofits (CalNonprofits)
Website: calnonprofits.org
Phone: (415) 777-1320

California Association of REALTORS (C.A.R.)
Website: car.org
Phone: (213) 739-8200

California Building Industry Association (CBIA)
Website: cbia.org
Phone: (916) 444-4300

Center for Sustainable Energy (CSE), California
Website: energycenter.org
Phone: (858) 244-1177

California Coalition for Rural Housing (CCRH)
Website: ccrh.org
Phone: (916) 447-2117

California Council for Environmental and Economic Balance (CCEEB)
Website: cceeb.org
Phone: (916) 444-2134

California Department of Community Services and Development (CSD)
Website: csd.ca.gov
Phone: (916) 576-7100

California Department of Housing and Community Development (HCD)
Website: hcd.ca.gov
Phone: (916) 445-4740

California Department of Public Health (CDPH)
Website: cdph.ca.gov
Phone: (916) 558-1784

California Department of Real Estate (DRE)
Website: dre.ca.gov
Phone: (877) 373-4542

California Department of Transportation (Caltrans)
Website: dot.ca.gov
Phone: (916) 654-2852

California Environmental Protection Agency (CalEPA)
Website: calepa.ca.gov
Phone: (916) 324-7870

Governor's Office of Business and Economic Development (GO-Biz)
Website: business.ca.gov
Phone: (916) 322-0694

California Homebuilding Foundation (CHF)

Website: chfoundation.org
Phone: (916) 448-8000

California Housing Finance Agency (CalHFA)
Website: calhfa.ca.gov
Phone: (916) 322-3991

California Housing Law Project
Website: housinglaw.org
Phone: (415) 703-8644

California Housing Partnership
Website: chpc.net
Phone: (415) 433-6804

California Land Title Association (CLTA)
Website: clta.org
Phone: (916) 444-2000

League of California Cities
Website: cacities.org
Phone: (916) 658-8200

California Natural Resources Agency
Website: resources.ca.gov
Phone: (916) 653-5656

Office of Statewide Health Planning and Development (OSHPD)
Website: oshpd.ca.gov
Phone: (916) 326-3800

California Redevelopment Association (CRA)
Website: calredevelop.org
Phone: (916) 448-8760

State Water Resources Control Board / Regional Water Boards
Website: waterboards.ca.gov
Phone: (916) 341-5254

California Society of Municipal Finance Officers (CSMFO)
Website: csmfo.org
Phone: (916) 231-2146

California State Association of Counties (CSAC)
Website: counties.org
Phone: (916) 327-7500

Contractors State License Board (CSLB), California
Website: cslb.ca.gov
Phone: (800) 321-2752

California Statewide Communities Development Authority (CSCDA)
Website: cscda.org
Phone: (916) 651-9790

Design-Build Institute of America (DBIA)
Website: dbia.org
Phone: (202) 682-0110

U.S. Economic Development Administration (EDA)
Website: eda.gov
Phone: (202) 482-4681

Housing California
Website: housingca.org
Phones: (916) 287-2947, (916) 447-0503

Mental Health Services Oversight and Accountability Commission (MHSOAC)
Website: mhsoac.ca.gov
Phone: (916) 445-8696

National Alliance on Mental Illness (NAMI) California
Website: namica.org
Phone: (916) 567-0163

National Housing Law Project (NHLP)
Website: nhlp.org
Phone: (415) 546-7000

San Diego Housing Federation
Website: housingsandiego.org
Phone: (619) 239-6693

40.U.S. Department of Housing and Urban Development (HUD) - California offices
Website: hud.gov/states/california/offices
Phone: Varies by regional office.

www.ingramcontent.com/pod-product-compliance
Lightning Source LLC
LaVergne TN
LVHW070945210926
848482LV00002B/105
9798900022369